MW00745565

MANUAL OF EMERGENCY ORTHOPAEDICS

PHILLIP M. SEGELOV
MB BS FRCS FRCSE FRACS

Consultant Orthopaedic Surgeon,
The Liverpool Hospital;

Senior Orthopaedic Surgeon,
Fairfield District Hospital;

Consultant Orthopaedic Surgeon,
St. George Hospital Skills Laboratory

FOREWORD BY
ERIC CASPARY
MB BS FRACS

Visiting Orthopaedic Surgeon
Fairfield District Hospital

Churchill Livingstone ▦

Edinburgh London Melbourne and New York 1986

CHURCHILL LIVINGSTONE
Medical Division of Longman
Group UK Limited

Distributed in the United States of
America by Churchill Livingstone
Inc., 1560 Broadway, New York,
N.Y. 10036, and by associated
companies, branches and
representatives throughout the
world.

© Longman Group UK Limited
1986

First published 1986

ISBN 0 443 03341 2

British Library Cataloguing in
Publication Data

Segelov, Phillip M.
    Manual of emergency orthopaedics.
    1. Orthopedia   2. Emergency
    medicine
    I. Title
    617′.3 RD732

Library of Congress Cataloging in
Publication Data

Segelov, Philip M.
    Manual of emergency orthopaedics.

    1. Orthopaedic emergencies.
    I. Title. [DNLM:
    1. Emergencies—handbooks.
    2. Orthopedics—handbooks.
    WE 39 S454m]
    RD750.S44
    1986 617′.1026 86-17182

Printed and bound in Great Britain by William Clowes Limited, Beccles and London

For Marise
and my children

FOREWORD

'Been there—done that!' could have been the alternative title of this manual. It is the favourite expression of the author, Phillip Segelov, who holds a unique place in the orthopaedic history of Australia. His dynamic personality has led him to the forefront in the practice, teaching, organisation and politics of orthopaedics in this country.

As the first person in Australia to practise advanced methods of internal fixation of fractures, initially his work was criticised. However, his results speak for themselves. He was made a member of AO International in honour of his work and has seen most Australian orthopaedic surgeons adopt these techniques.

At the age of fifty, a myocardial infarct slowed him down for long enough to begin a long term ambition—a manual for hospital housemen.

Written in the old style, it suffers the advantages and disadvantages of single man authorship. No double-blind trials followed by half a dozen possible methods of treatment here! It is simply full of advice from a senior surgeon based on twenty-five years of experience. The book contains many illustrations with brief and occasionally abrupt summaries—you may well be talking to the author direct. Most of the common and major casualty orthopaedic problems can be located by X-ray or diagram. While written for the less experienced, some orthopaedic surgeons in training may find it useful.

We hope, that as time goes on and the owner of this manual calls on it less and less, when confronted with an orthopaedic problem he or she will look up at the book on the shelf and be able to say: 'Been there—done that!'

Eric Caspary

PREFACE

This book is designed to help the Casualty Officer identify orthopaedic or fracture problems that he or she may come across, and to offer the correct primary treatment. There are often many ways a problem can be handled; this book does not pretend to cover them all. It is *not* an orthopaedic textbook and thus rare and unusual conditions are not included.

This manual started as a few pages of notes, and grew as a result of requests from the people it is now intended to help–the young and inexperienced Casualty Officer.

No book is written without help from many sources. My thanks are due to John Cumming for the artwork, to Bill Miles for finding all those X-rays and to my partner, Eric Caspary, for his advice and criticism. My thanks are also due to my publishers for the monumental task of advising a novice.

1986   P.M.S.

CONTENTS

CHAPTER ONE

Fractures: general introduction

General remarks

By definition a fracture is a break in the continuity of a bone and the most tender spot is usually the site of the fracture. The classical signs of a fracture — pain, swelling, loss of function, and crepitus — may not be present in a greenstick (Fig. 1.1) or incomplete fracture, but in a displaced fracture not only do we have the signs mentioned but of course there is also deformity.

It is axiomatic that you X-ray all suspected fractures.

Do I have it X-rayed tonight?

Can I justify calling in a radiographer after hours?

The answer to these questions depends on you asking yourself the following:

Is this likely to be a fracture or not?

If it is a fracture is it likely to need reduction tonight?

Remember that provided you immobilise a fracture and give analgesics most simple fractures can be left overnight.

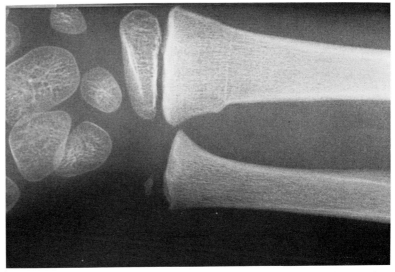

Fig. 1.1 Greenstick fracture of the distal radius.

You must immobilise with a padded plaster backslab and warn the patient and/or the parents that if they have severe pain or circulation problems they are to return to casualty.

Please order X-rays that include the joint above and below the tender area.

Looking at X-rays

It is of the utmost importance that the doctor should be able to interpret an X-ray correctly. He needs to decide if a fracture is present and if it is displaced. Does it need reduction?

The first step is to see that the X-rays are on the viewing box the correct way up! Make sure that they are the correct X-rays and that the left side is on the *left* and in the case of a wrist that the thumb metacarpal is pointing to the floor. If you fail to do this, you will mistake a Smith's fracture (Fig. 1.2) for a Colles' fracture (Fig. 1.3).

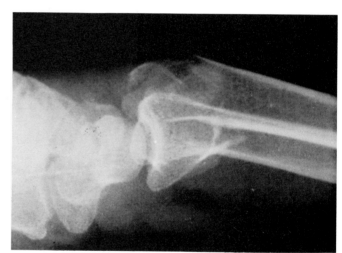

Fig. 1.2   Smith's fracture.

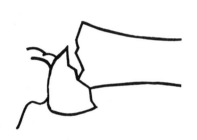

Fig. 1.3   Colles' fracture.

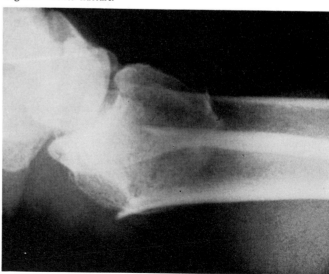

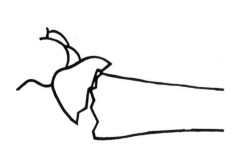

The next thing is to be sure that you can see on the X-rays the joint above and below the suspect area and that there is not a second injury such as a fracture or dislocation that you are missing. The classic mistake is to miss a dislocated hip when the patient has a fractured femur (Fig. 1.4).

Always think and describe displacement of the distal fragment on the proximal — thus a Colles' fracture is displaced dorsally and radially and is often impacted.

Angulation is described according to where the apex of the fracture points.

Displacement is described according to which way the distal fragment is pushed on the proximal one.

It is always necessary to have both an antero-posterior and a lateral view. Sometimes oblique views are also necessary.

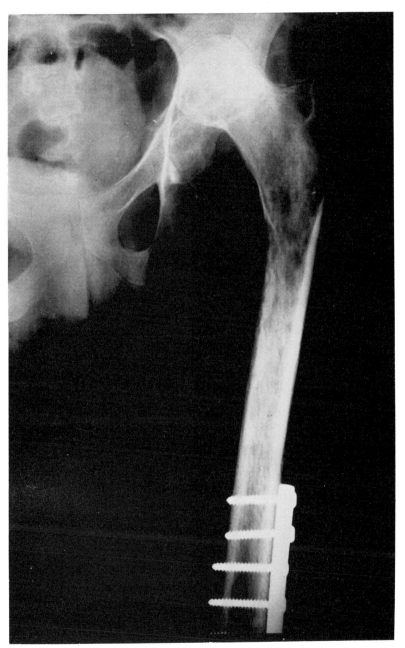

Fig. 1.4 The fractured femur has been plated, but the dislocated hip was missed.

Children's X-rays can be difficult to interpret, particularly around the elbow joint and at the wrist, due to the epiphyses that appear at differing ages. Some help is always there because you can X-ray the opposite elbow or wrist for comparison. Epiphyses are the same on both sides and of course are not tender if not injured. In addition, a fracture is jagged and irregular, whereas an epiphysis is rounded and smooth.

Look at the alignment of the epiphysis to be certain that there is not displacement of the epiphysis as a whole and compare it with the other side.

The elbow is the most difficult region in children as there are multiple epiphyses and they appear at different ages — be careful of the epiphysis of the medial epicondyle in a dislocated elbow in a child, it is commonly avulsed and may be in the joint. Look carefully at what can happen to the epiphysis of the medial epicondyle (Fig. 1.5).

Fig. 1.5   Various types of displacement of the medial epicondyle.

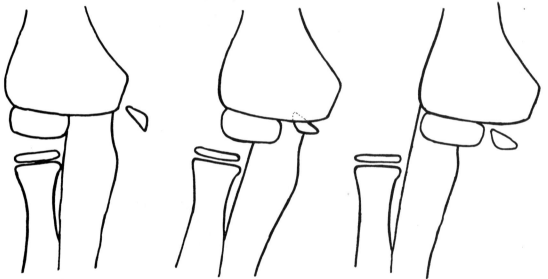

Does the fracture need reduction?

You will need to see the discussion of each fracture to decide this but here are some rules to help:

1. Fractures involving joints (Fig. 1.6) or epiphyses (Fig. 1.7) must be accurately reduced and often require open reduction.

2. Displacement of up to fifty per cent of the width of the bone can be accepted in one or more planes provided there is no angulation or rotation.

3. In an adult (Figs. 1.8 and .1.9) all shortening, angulation and rotation should, if possible, be corrected in the lower limb — even if open reduction becomes necessary.

4. In a child, nature will often come to our aid and will correct the angulation and deformity with growth. Remember the younger the child the more correction will occur and the faster it occurs. The closer the deformity is to the epiphysis, the faster the correction. In an eight year old, thirty degrees of correction will be complete within about nine months if the injury is within one

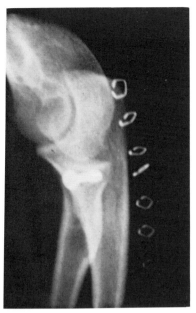

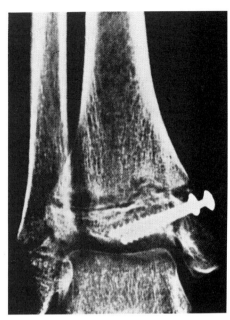

Fig. 1.6 Postoperative X-ray of a fractured head of radius.

Fig. 1.7 Postoperative X-ray of an epiphyseal fracture of the ankle.

Fig. 1.8 Angulated fracture of the tibia and fibula.

Fig. 1.9 Angulated, shortened and rotated fracture of the tibia and fibula.

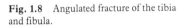

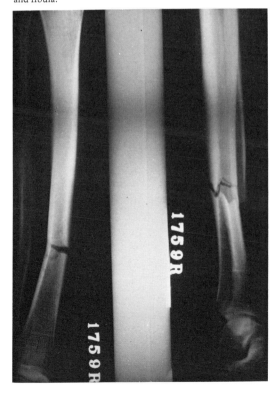

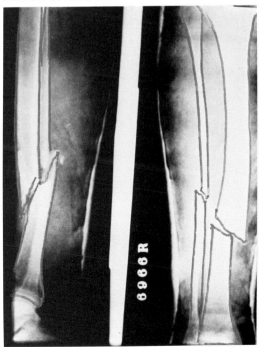

Fig. 1.10 (a) Fracture of the neck of the humerus in a child of eight. (b) The same fracture four weeks later, showing early moulding.

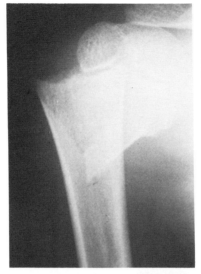
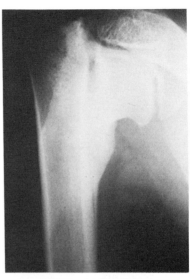

centimetre of the epiphysis (Fig. 1.10).

There is very little correction of deformity in the upper limb after the age of eleven and in the lower limb after the age of fourteen.

5. Remember you are not treating an X-ray or even a fracture but a person with a fracture that has been X-rayed. There may well be good reason for accepting the position of a fracture that is otherwise unsatisfactory. The fracture shown in Figure 1.11 is acceptable in a very frail old lady but not in a healthy young person.

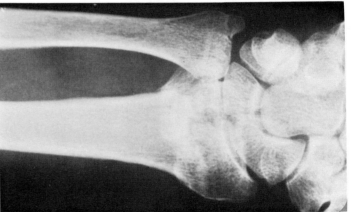

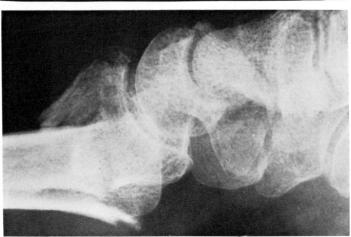

Fig. 1.11 (a) Antero-posterior X-ray of a Colles' fracture. (b) Lateral X-ray of a Colles' fracture..

How to reduce a fracture

Please see each individual fracture for details. Here are some general hints:

1. Examine the X-rays closely and be sure in your own mind which way the fragments are displaced.

2. **When the patient is anaesthetized** pick up the limb and feel the fracture site gently — most bones can be palpated easily through the soft tissues — make sure that you can feel the deformity that you can see on the X-rays. If you are in doubt then go back to the X-rays until you are sure.

3. Now you are ready to reduce the fracture. Most fractures require traction to overcome the shortening and then direct pressure over the displaced distal fragment — a lot more force is required than most people think. Use the intact periosteum on one side of the fracture to help you as shown in Figure 1.12.

4. Run your finger along the line of the bone and over the fracture site. If it is reduced, then the bump at the fracture site that you had previously palpated should have disappeared. To be sure of this **gently** displace the fracture again and recreate the deformity, then palpate it and reduce — this way, you can be sure in your own mind that it is reduced. **Use your fingers as your guide** and only X-ray the fracture when it is reduced.

5. You are now ready to apply plaster slabs as outlined below. This is where the reduction of many fractures is lost — care needs to be taken by the person holding the limb to maintain the position and in forearm fractures you are better leaving the limb hanging because an assistant picking up the hand will displace the distal fragment.

Fig. 1.12 (a) The periosteal hinge and (b) how it is used in fracture reduction.

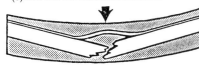

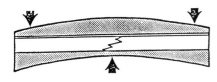

Circulatory problems

The last thing you need is to create problems for yourself and for the patient by either ignoring a threat to the circulation or by creating one. It takes but a second to check the circulation in fingers and toes and to show the parents how to do this. If a patient has a displaced ankle fracture or a supracondylar fracture of the humerus then check the circulation **immediately** on arrival in Casualty — if it is deficient give some analgesic and pull on the limb so as to align the fracture a little better even before X-rays are done. In almost all cases, the circulation will return when the gross deformity has been reduced and will thereafter be no problem.

If the circulation does not return, you must advise the consultant immediately.

Do not put a full plaster on a recent fracture

Since adopting this rule, twenty-five years ago, we have not had a single case of Volkmann's ischaemic contracture or circulatory troubles due to tight plaster. There are a few cases where a full plaster may be necessary, then **the plaster and padding must be fully split.**

Do not put a full plaster on a recent fracture

Backslabs or back and side slabs so that the limb is supported on about two-thirds of its circumference are the ideal way to immobilize a recent fracture. Some padding is applied and then the slabs are held on by firm but not tight crepe bandages. This means that there is room for swelling and that when the patient is seen at the one week stage it is easy to tighten the slabs with Elastoplast or to complete the plaster. It is also easy to remove the plaster by cutting through the soft bandage.

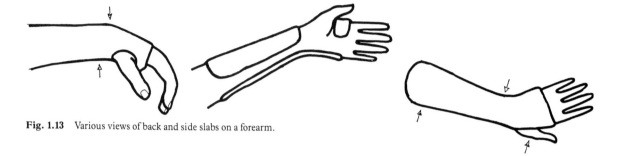

Fig. 1.13 Various views of back and side slabs on a forearm.

Use backslabs and sideslabs

Remember that a backslab (Fig. 1.13) will protect the fracture site from being knocked whether the arms is by the side or in a sling. The fracture site is painful, so it is important to protect the area from being hit by a passerby.

Compound fractures

The magic word 'compound' applied to fractures causes many a muttered swear word amongst orthopaedic surgeons since they are usually caused by the folly of a car driver or a motor bike rider.

Think a little. A compound fracture is a fracture in communication with the air. Is there a difference between a minor puncture wound from within and a massive crushing and dirty wound (each with a fracture)?

Of course there is. A much more sensible approach would grade the fracture and describe the following.

1. *The bone* — The site of the fracture, the joint involvement and comminution.

2. *The wound* — The size and situation, the involvement of nerves and vessels and is it a crushing wound or more of a cut?

3. *The contamination* — How dirty is the wound? Wounds from within are basically clean.

4. *The mechanism of injury* — A high velocity injury, a crushing injury, or just a simple fall with a compound wound from within.

In Casualty **for all compound fractures** you must do the following:

1. Assess the patient as a whole. Be aware that the compound injury may be the obvious injury, **but not the only one.** Check the patient for abdominal and pelvic injuries and monitor the pulse and blood pressure.

2. Set up a drip and give the patient some intravenous antibiotics. What you use, depends on the choice at your hospital. We are currently using one of the cephalosporins for non-allergic patients.

3. Give the patient adequate analgesia (intravenously for rapid action) according to age and size but avoid if possible when there are

head injuries and before assessment of abdominal injuries.

4. Tetanus toxoid or TIg is given according to whether the patient is immunised. (See section on *Tetanus prophylaxis* below.)

5. Examine the wound and grade the injury in the terms mentioned above. Remember to reapply the compression dressing and splinting.

6. Arrange X-rays, notify consultants and arrange the operating theatre.

The next steps depend on the severity of the injury (grading).

Grade 1: Minor compound fractures. The compound element is small and the contamination minimal. The wound (Fig. 1.14) can be dealt with in casualty. Clean the wound, which in this grade can only be a puncture wound or a small cut. The fracture (Fig. 1.15) is dealt with on its merits, by closed or open reduction as though there was no wound.

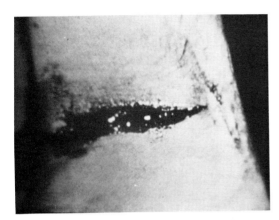

Fig. 1.14 Clean, non-contaminated, wound over a tibial fracture.

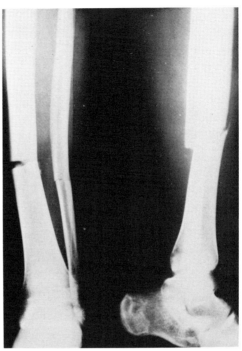

Fig. 1.15 X-ray of the fracture of the tibia and fibula occurring with the wound shown in Figure 1.14.

Fig. 1.16 A severe contaminated wound with much tissue damage.

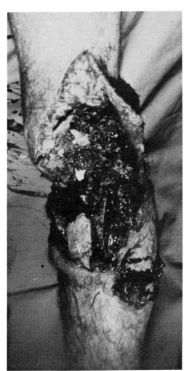

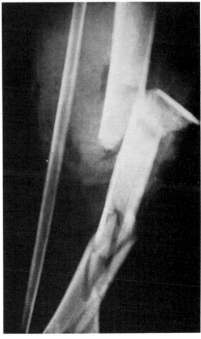

Grades 2, 3 and 4: Serious compound fractures. For the casualty officer, all the grades above the first will involve him or her in the initial management only because the definitive primary treatment, which will include debridement and repair and reduction of the fracture, will all take place in the operating theatre (Figs. 1.16 and 1.17).

You will need to arrange blood for transfusion in the more serious compound fractures, and of course restoration of blood volume and blood pressure is essential in these patients, before debridement and treatment of the fracture.

Fig. 1.17 The fracture associated with the wound shown in Figure 1.16.

Severe bleeding

Sometimes in association with a compound fracture or a large wound, blood gushes forth from the patient at an alarming rate. What do you do?

Don't panic as almost all bleeding can be stopped by a combination of direct pressure and elevation:

1. Apply a large pad or pads and if the bleeding is from a wound on a limb, then a very firm bandage should be applied. If necessary, put another pad and another bandage on it.

2. Elevate the limb.

3. Start up a drip to replace the lost circulatory volume and organize blood cross matching.

4. If there is still a lot of bleeding, then direct pressure by hand over the wound is your next step.

5. If bleeding is still not controlled, an arterial tourniquet is your next step. Use a blood pressure cuff or pneumatic tourniquet, make sure that it is pumped up above the blood pressure and does not make things worse by being a venous tourniquet.

You will need help from a more experienced colleague especially if this is a main artery and it has to be repaired.

6. Your patient will need strong analgesia if an arterial tourniquet is to be left on for more than a few minutes and you must arrange immediate repair as the limb **is devoid of blood supply** whilst the arterial tourniquet is on. The patient may not be bleeding to death but the limb is dying!

Do not use artery forceps unless the situation is such that no other measure will stop the bleeding. By clamping the end of an important artery you may make direct repair impossible due to the crushing of the artery wall.

7. Once the bleeding is under control and the patient has been transfused, definitive treatment can be arranged.

8. **Do not remove large penetrating foreign bodies in Casualty — you may start torrential bleeding from deep within the wound.**

Tetanus prophylaxis

Prophylactic tetanus toxoid or TIg (Tetanus immunoglobulin — Human) should be given in all compound fractures and indeed in all significant wounds as follows:

(a) Fully immunized patient. If more than one year has elapsed since last dose, give a booster dose of toxoid.

(b) Non-immune or partially-immune patient — give TIg plus a dose of toxoid at a different site. TIg, 250 international units, is normally given i.m. but in severe contamination give 500 i.u.

(c) Complete the course of immunization with further doses of toxoid.

TIg circulates in the body at an effective dose for at least four weeks.

Gas gangerene serum is seldom used as it is felt to be of doubtful efficacy. It is much more important for wounds to be adequately debrided and left open, and for adequate or large doses of i.v. penicillin (or other antibiotics if the patient is allergic to penicillin) to be given in such cases.

ATS (antitetanus serum) is a bovine or equine preparation and has no indication now that TIg is available.

Anaesthesia and analgesia

Whilst full anaesthesia (either regional or general) is necessary for most severely displaced fractures, those with angulation or minor displacement that simply require a push can be dealt with after an appropriate dose (for age and size) of pethidine and diazepam (Valium).

Remember that we must not torture our patients and this latter form of treatment must be reserved for those fractures that can be put back into place with *one* push. If multiple pushes and pulls are required, then one of the following methods of anaesthesia must be used:

Intravenous local anaesthesia with tourniquet

This is a useful technique, especially in a patient who has eaten recently, and should be mastered by all casualty officers. It involves applying a tourniquet after exsanguinating the limb and then injecting an appropriate amount of lignocaine into the vein through a scalp vein cannula.

The local anaesthetic diffuses from the vein and gives excellent analgesia in the region. The tourniquet should be kept elevated for ten minutes. Accidental release of the tourniquet may cause a fall in blood pressure and possibly convulsions if the dosage has been high and if the local anaesthetic has not been fixed by the tissues.

Fixation of a local anaesthetic is rapid and I have used this technique hundreds of times without problems.

Details:
1. Give some sedation, as necessary
2. Measure blood pressure and record
3. Insert two butterfly i.v. cannulae. One in the back of the hand or dorsum of the foot and **a second one, for emergencies, in the other hand**
4. Exsanguinate the limb using a rubber bandage, **or elevate if too painful**
5. **Use a proper pneumatic orthopaedic tourniquet, not a blood pressure cuff, as they are unreliable**
6. Inflate the **tourniquet** to be 50 mmHG **above** the patient's systolic blood pressure
7. **Inject 0.6 ml of 0.05 per cent plain lignocaine per kg of body weight (maximum amount 50 ml)**
8. Wait a few minutes and then proceed
9. Leave tourniquet on for a minimum of ten minutes
10. **Do not use MARCAINE (fatalities have occurred)**
11. **Always have oxygen and resuscitation cart available**

Local anaesthesia into the fracture

This effectively converts a simple fracture into a compound fracture and since abscesses and dirty wounds are dressed in most casualty departments, I do not think that this technique should be used.

Local nerve block

In this technique, a small amount of local is injected into the appropriate nerve trunks. It is a valuable one and is quite easy provided you know where the appropriate nerve trunks are hidden. It is particularly helpful in finger injuries where a digital block will enable you to repair soft tissues and to reduce any fractures of the phalanges. It can be used for forearm fractures by blocking the nerve trunks of the three nerves around the elbow. The use of a femoral nerve block in fractures of the femur allows you to apply traction and reduce the fracture without distressing the patient.

Digital nerve block

Each digit is supplied by four nerve branches, two on the dorsal aspect and two on the palmar aspect. A total of 1.0 to 2.0 ml of 1 per cent lignocaine needs to be injected around each nerve (Fig. 1.18) and across the dorsal and vental aspects to catch any branches of the nerves.

Do not use local anaesthetic with ADRENALINE (EPINEPHRINE) in fingers, toes or penis as their arteries are end-arteries and gangrene of the digit or penis may occur. Also avoid large volumes of local anaesthetic agent.

Fig. 1.18 Technique of digital nerve block. **N.B. No adrenaline (epinephrine) in the local anaesthetic.**

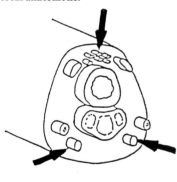

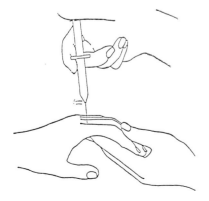

Femoral nerve block

This is a valuable block for the casualty officer to know because it is an excellent way to control pain in a fracture of the femur (in both children and adults) whilst you are putting the patient up in traction.

Anatomy (Fig. 1.19)

The femoral nerve enters the anterior part of the thigh by passing deep to the inguinal ligament, lying on the psoas muscle and lateral to

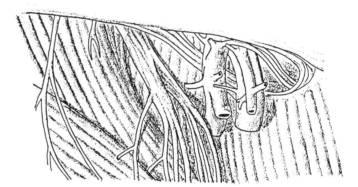

Fig. 1.19 Anatomy of inguinal region.

the femoral artery. The nerve divides into two bundles usually just below the inguinal ligament, but occasionally above the ligament. The anterior bundle innervates the skin of the anteror aspect of the thigh and the sartorius muscle. The posterior group innervates the quadriceps muscles, the knee joint, and gives off the saphenous nerve.

Technique

Block the femoral nerve immediately below the inguinal ligament. Palpate the femoral artery and insert a fine needle lateral to the

vessel to a depth of 3.5 cm (Fig. 1.20). The needle may pulsate. If you do penetrate the artery, apply compression for 10 minutes to prevent haematoma formation.

20 ml of 1 per cent lignocaine with adrenaline is injected in a fan shaped area from the original depth to the subcutaneous level and out laterally to a point about 3 cm from the artery.

Sometimes, whilst you are injecting the lignocaine, the patient complains of parasthesiae. If they

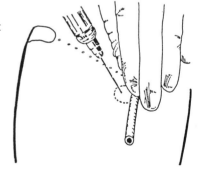

Fig. 1.20 Technique of femoral nerve block.

do, then inject 10 ml at that point, but continue the fan shaped injection as the nerve may well have already divided.

CHAPTER TWO

Fractures of the upper limb

Phalanges of the hand

One of the more common injuries seen in the casualty section of any hospital are fractures of the phalanges. The principles of management are the same in adults and children, except that in children there are two additional factors to be considered — an advantage and a disadvantage.

Advantage. The child's ability to recover from damage to a joint and regain more movement than one would expect and a limited ability to mould deformity with growth.

Disadvantage. The possibility of partial or complete growth cessation, if an epiphyseal plate is damaged by a fracture.

Simple fractures (i.e. non-compound)

These fractures are still problems if they fall in the 'movement zone' of the hand (Fig. 2.1). Any fracture in this area can result in stiffness and deformity if not properly handled.

Fig. 2.1 'Movement Zone' of hand.

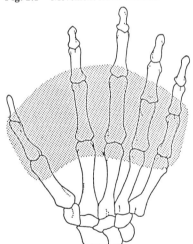

1. Recognize the fracture by having any significant injury X-rayed. When viewing the films, pay particular attention to the very tender areas.

2. Undisplaced fractures require splinting of the hand in 'the position of function' (Fig. 2.2). This can be done simply with a strip of padded aluminium splinting material bent into shape. **'The position of function' is the position that the hand falls into as you relax your hand.**

Fig. 2.2 'Position of function' of the hand.

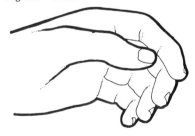

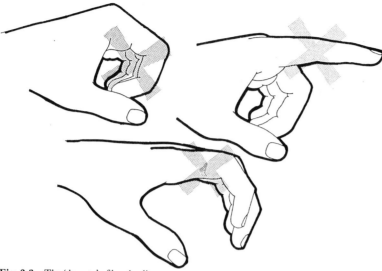

Fig. 2.3 The 'do nots' of hand splintage:
(a) Not fully flexed; **(b)** Not out straight;
and **(c)** Not clawed.

**Do not splint fingers out
straight** with all joints extended
(Fig. 2.3) because the ligaments are
tight in extension and as they
contract with splinting the whole
finger will become stiff.

**Do not splint the fingers fully
flexed (Fig. 2.3)**

**Do not splint the hand 'clawed'
(Fig. 2.3)**
It is often a good idea to splint an
adjacent finger to the injured one to
prevent rotation and angulation.

4. A **displaced** fracture will
require reduction and this will need
to be done perfectly, especially in
relation to angulation and rotation.
A finger that is angulated and
rotated just cannot bend in concert
with the other fingers (Fig. 2.4).

5. The technique of reduction is
shown in Figure 2.5. To prevent
slipping and to give greater traction
you can put some Elastoplast on the
end of the finger. These fractures
can be managed best with a regional
anaesthesia (described in the *Digital
nerve block* section, Chapter 1).

Traction should be in the line of
the finger and rotation can easily be
checked by observing the position of
the fingernail (Fig. 2.4).

It is often advisable to reduce the
overlap to gain end to end
apposition and then to apply the
splint. When the finger is on the
splint, then correct the angulation
and rotation.

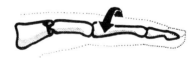

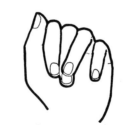

Fig. 2.4   Rotational deformity in finger
fractures.

Fig. 2.5   Method of reduction of a
fractured phalanx.

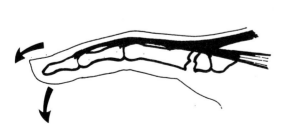

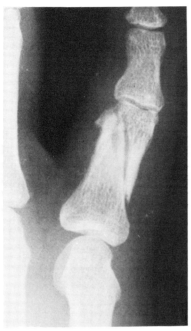

Unless the position of the fracture is perfect open reduction may be necessary (Fig. 2.6).
Reduction and fixation using percutaneous K-wires is the technique that is often used (Figs. 2.7 and 2.8).

Fig. 2.6 Spiral fracture of proximal phalanx with shortening.

Fig. 2.7 Intra-articular fracture of the base of the distal phalanx.

Fig. 2.8 A fine longitudonal K-wire holding a fracture of the distal end of the middle phalanx in a good position.

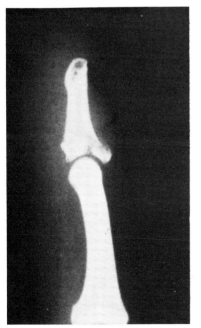

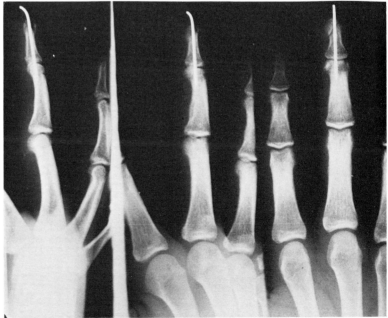

Fractures that involve the joints (Figs. 2.9 and 2.10) require special care to ensure that the joint surfaces are restored as much as possible either by open (Fig. 2.10) or closed methods (Figs. 2.11a and b). Thus the stability and the gliding surface of the joints are left in the best possible state.

Some of the many sites of fractures of the phalanges are shown in Figure 2.12.

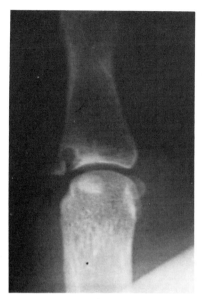

Fig. 2.9   Fracture of the base of the proximal phalanx of the thumb, an avulsion injury − note the rotation of the fragment.

Fig. 2.10   The lateral view of the thumb in Figure 2.9.

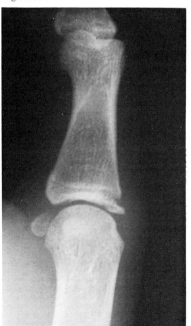

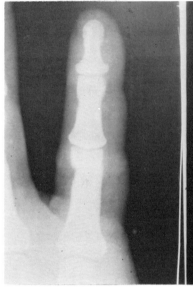
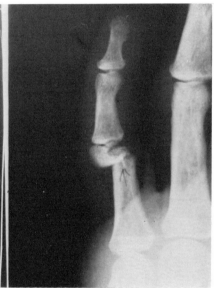

Fig. 2.11(a)   Fracture of the distal end of the proximal phalanx of an index finger with displacement and rotation.

Fig. 2.11(b)   The same fracture as in (a) after reduction and splinting.

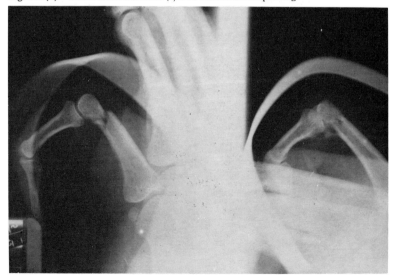

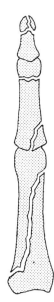

Fig. 2.12 Common sites of phalangeal fractures.

Distal phalanx — distal tuft

Ouch! Every time I see a fractured distal phalanx I can almost feel the hammer hitting the fingertip. This is the common way this fracture occurs (Fig. 2.13a). This fracture itself is not really a problem as there is often minimal displacement *but* it is really painful because this is an area well supplied with sensation. Thus, unless the fracture is compound through the nail bed, the haematoma that forms is tense and painful.

Figs. 2.13(a) and **(b)** Bursting fracture of the distal phalanx; and **(c)** how it occurs.

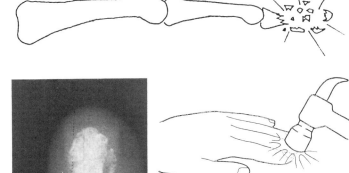

Treatment

1. Simple fractures of the distal phalanx (Fig. 2.13) require a short protective splint of padded aluminium bent up over the end of the finger.

2. If the haematoma is tense and throbbing, open and drain the haematoma. This can be done in any of three ways:

   (a) Drill a hole in the nail with a heated needle

   (b) Drill a hole gently with a very pointed scalpel

   (c) Lift the nail fold off the nail with a scalpel

Apply a bulky dressing — you can incorporate a short length of aluminium splint bent over the distal phalanx to protect the tender area.

3. Compound wounds with blood oozing from the nail bed, or from crushed soft tissue in the pulp of the finger, will require cleaning and dressing with a non-adherent gauze and then a padded dressing. Since it is a bursting type wound sutures are usually contra-indicated and the fracture itself is usually ignored. Antibiotics will be necessary and the dressing should be changed in two days, before it becomes caked with blood and hard. When the wound has healed, careful use of the finger can be started, but the fingertip will remain sore for about twelve weeks.

A common injury in children is the fracture of the base of the fourth or fifth proximal phalanx involving the epiphysis with **ulnar (medial) deviation** (Fig. 2.14). **The injury is best treated by splinting the injured finger or fingers to the adjacent uninjured finger** (Fig. 2.15). This not only corrects the alignment but allows for a **mobile splint,** the other finger. Splint the finger for three weeks.

Mallet finger (Fig. 2.16) is dealt with in the chapter on *Tendon injuries* (Ch. 6).

Dislocations of the finger joints are dealt with in the chapter on *Dislocations* (Ch. 5).

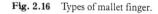
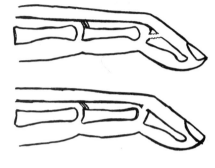

Fig. 2.16　Types of mallet finger.

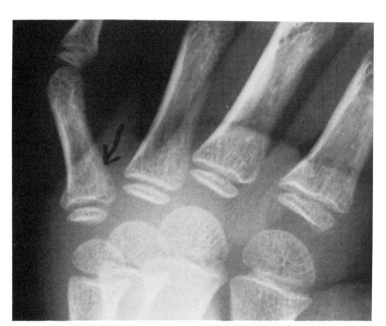

Fig. 2.14　Fracture of the base of the proximal phalanx little finger, in a child.

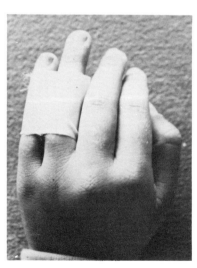

Fig. 2.15　Reduction and 'mobile splinting' of the fracture shown in Figure 2.14.

Metacarpals

A fall on the hand, a punch that hits something hard, or a heavy object that falls on the hand, are the usual causes of this injury which can occur at any age. These fractures can occur at the base, in the shaft, or at the neck of the metacarpal bone (Fig. 2.17).

However a simple splint (Fig. 2.18) or backslab can be applied for comfort and kept on for a few weeks if the patient finds the fracture painful. Mostly patients abandon the splint or backslab after a few days and then begin active exercises with care.

Fig. 2.18(a)   Simple splinting using a padded aluminium strip; and **(b)** followed by active exercises.

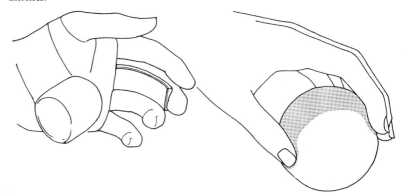

Fig. 2.17   Sites of fracture in the metacarpal bones.

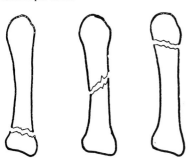

Undisplaced fractures are well splinted by the adjacent metacarpal bone (or bones) and their attached ligaments and muscles.

The displaced fracture is rare and will require reduction. If it is unstable, then a K-wire through the adjacent metacarpal (Fig. 2.19) will be sufficient to hold it in place. This must be done in the operating theatre, under X-ray or image intensifier control to see that the position is satisfactory. Your role in casualty will be to splint the hand for comfort and make the necessary arrangements. Displaced fractures are always more painful than undisplaced ones and analgesics will be needed.

Fig. 2.19(a)   Displaced fracture of metacarpal bone; and **(b)** horizontal K-wire fixation.

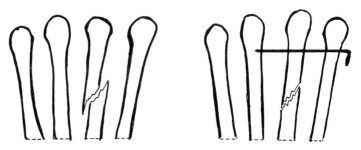

Metacarpal neck with angulation

This is very commonly the result of a missed punch — the victim ducks and the assailant hits the wall with his fist clenched and his wrist partly flexed. The metacarpal head takes the blow on the dorsal aspect of the bone, the metacarpal neck snaps and the head angulates into the palm (Fig. 2.20). Twenty to thirty per cent angulation can be accepted as

the metacarpal head has a very extensive articular surface. The net effect, as far as the patient is concerned, is that they lose the prominence of the knuckle when the fist is clenched but function in the hand is not impaired and provided you warn the patient of the minor cosmetic change they will be happy.

More severe angulation will

justify closed reduction under regional anaesthesia.

The method of reduction shown in Figure 2.21a, b depends on the piston effect of squeezing together the distal end of the proximal phalanx and the metacarpal proximal to the fracture.

Fig. 2.20   Fracture of the metacarpal neck with angulation.

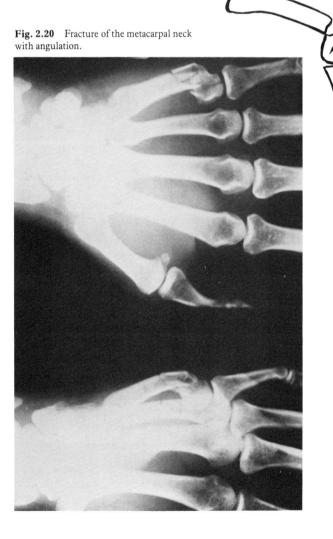

Fig. 2.21   Methods of reduction and splintage of fractures of the metacarpal neck.

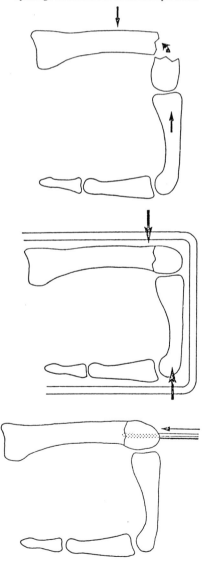

A bandage or an aluminium splint can be applied to the finger with it flexed in the 90 to 90 position. This extreme position should be changed after ten days (when the fracture is getting sticky) to the 'position of function'.

Open reduction is *only* necessary if there is complete separation of the head with displacement. Care is needed to prevent fixation in malrotation (Fig. 2.21c).

Bennett's fracture dislocation

Who was Bennett and why was this fracture dislocation named after him?

He was an anatomist at Trinity College Dublin who later became professor of surgery and president of the Royal College of Surgeons of Ireland. He was reputed to be a stimulating teacher, and a model of honour and uprightness who never did a crooked thing. He was blunt but not unkind. He described the injury in a paper in 1882 entitled, *Fractures of the metacarpal bones*.

Bennett's fracture dislocation usually occurs in adults following a violent extension force on the thumb (Fig. 2.22). It is a fracture of the base of the first metacarpal with joint involvement (Fig. 2.23) and usually dislocation of the thumb proximally under the strong pull of the flexors and extensors.

Note the site of fracture — it is just distal to the anatomical snuff box. The most common mistake is to think that the fracture is one joint distally at the thumb 'knuckle' (metacarpophalangeal joint).

Suspect a Bennett's fracture when there is pain, tenderness, bruising, occasionally palpable crepitus and instability of the base of the thumb.

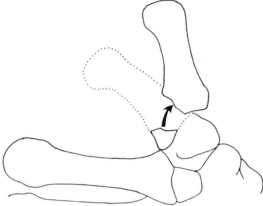

Fig. 2.22 The mechanics of a Bennett's fracture caused by a violent extension force on the thumb.

Fig. 2.23 X-ray of a Bennett's fracture with displacement.

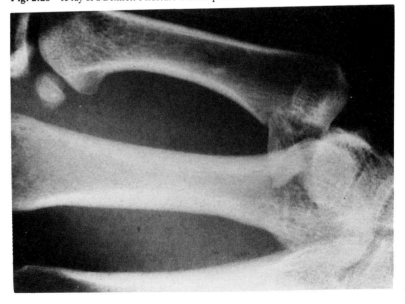

Management

Bennett's fracture is an intra-articular fracture (Fig. 2.24) and as such requires accurate anatomical reduction.

Closed reduction requires anaesthesia (general or regional), traction on the thumb and direct pressure over the metacarpal base whilst the plaster is setting (Fig. 2.25). The base of the metacarpal needs a piece of felt over it as padding.

Note that the thumb is not **abducted — it is adducted** and then the pressure is applied before the plaster sets (Fig. 2.25).

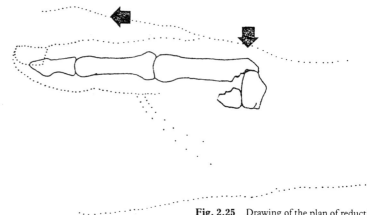

Fig. 2.25   Drawing of the plan of reduction of a Bennett's fracture, showing traction on the adducted thumb and direct pressure.

X-rays need to be taken post-reduction, and again in one week. If reduction is not satisfactory, or is not maintained, then open reduction needs to be done.

Fig. 2.24   Bennett's fracture is an intra-articular fracture with subluxation of most of the base of the thumb metacarpal.

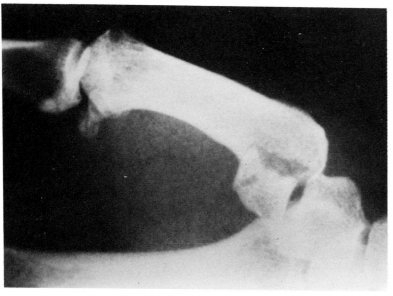

It is my practice to treat these fractures by percutaneous pinning under image intensifier control (Fig. 2.26) as reduction can be obtained, confirmed and maintained by pinning. The pins are left in place for five weeks and then removed in the consulting rooms without anaesthesia.

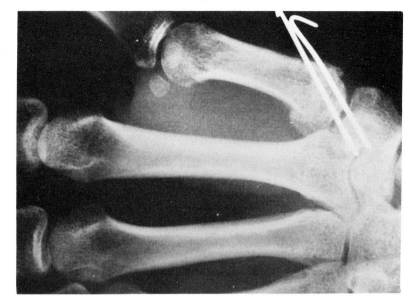

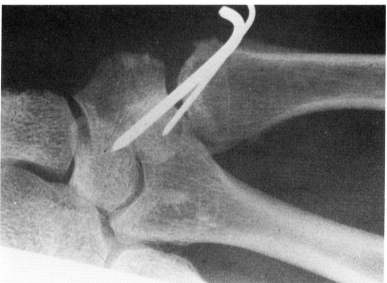

Fig. 2.26 Percutaneous pinning of Bennett's fracture.

Carpus — wrist

Carpal scaphoid

This is the fracture that is so often missed, as the scaphoid bone is (as its Latin name says) boat shaped and hence the initial fracture line, if not displaced, is hidden by overlying bone.

What can we do to avoid missing these fractures? There are four rules:

1. Suspect this fracture in any person who falls on the wrist and is tender in the anatomical snuff box (Fig. 2.27). Pressure along the index or ring finger will also cause pain (Fig. 2.28).

Fig. 2.27 Site of tenderness in a fractured scaphoid.

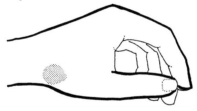

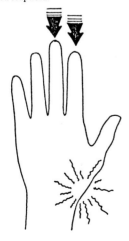

Fig. 2.28 Pressure over the end of the index and middle fingers causes pain in a fractured scaphoid.

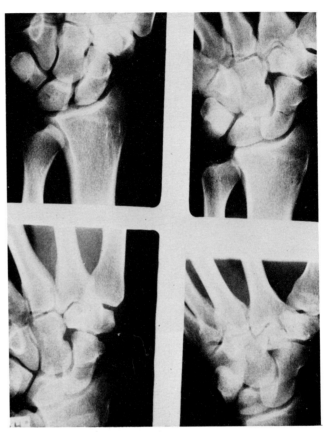

Fig. 2.29 'Scaphoid series' of X-rays for detection of scaphoid fractures.

2. X-ray these patients, not just with antero-posterior views but also with oblique views as in the 'scaphoid series' shown in Figure 2.29.

3. Even when the X-rays appear to show no fracture, if the area is very tender put the patient in plaster.

4. Take further X-rays in ten days, and even repeat a few weeks later if the soreness persists. Figure

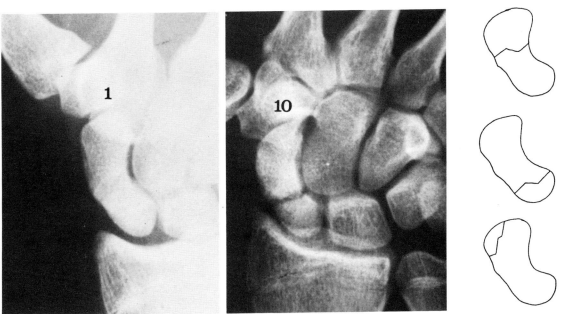

Fig. 2.30 Scaphoid X-rays at (a) one and (b) ten days, showing how easy it is to overlook this fracture on day one.

Fig. 2.32 Sites of fracture in the scaphoid bone.

2.30a shows a wrist injury and fractured scaphoid on day one. Figure 2.30b shows the same patient ten days later.

If untreated, the fracture of the waist of the scaphoid bone will not unite, and over a ten to fifteen year period a severe arthritis may develop in the wrist as is seen in the X-rays in Figure 2.31a and b.

Figure 2.32 shows three sites of fracture of the scaphoid bone.

Fig. 2.31(a) The early fractured scaphoid; and (b) the neglected fractured scaphoid – after 11 years, with arthritis between the scaphoid and the radius.

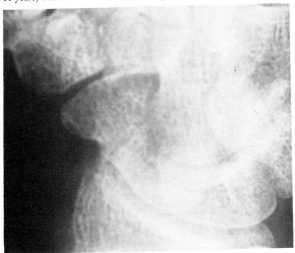

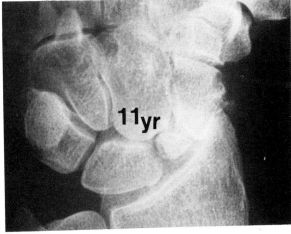

Management

All fractures of the scaphoid and
suspected fractures of the scaphoid
need to be immobilised in a
'scaphoid type' plaster. Note that
the plaster includes the thumb
distally to the interphalangeal joint
(Figs. 2.33 and 2.34), and that the
hand is in the 'ball holding position'.
As the plaster will be on for some
time, use a waterproof plastic
splinting material (Fig. 2.33) instead
of plaster (Fig. 2.34).

   Displaced fractures of the
scaphoid may require reduction and
even internal fixation (Fig. 2.35),
whilst old fractures will not unite
with simple plaster immobilization.

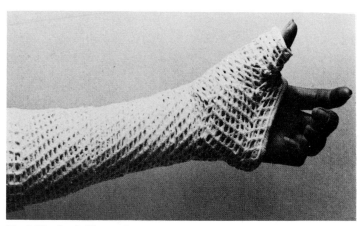

Fig. 2.33   Scaphoid type of waterproof plastic 'plaster'.

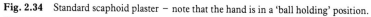

Fig. 2.34   Standard scaphoid plaster – note that the hand is in a 'ball holding' position.

Fig. 2.35   Internal fixation of a fractured
scaphoid using a Herbert screw.

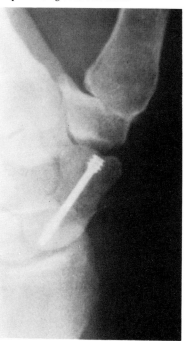

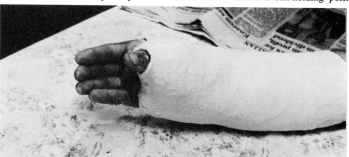

Is it an old fracture? An old
fracture (Fig. 2.36a) has a wider gap
and the edges of the fracture are
rounded and not sharp and jagged as
in a recent fracture (Fig. 2.36b).

   How long does it have to stay in
plaster?

   Three weeks for a fracture of the
tuberosity (Fig. 2.37).

   Six weeks for a fracture of the
waist (Fig. 2.38), and then X-ray and
assess clinically. A further four
weeks in plaster is often necessary.

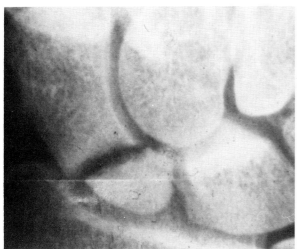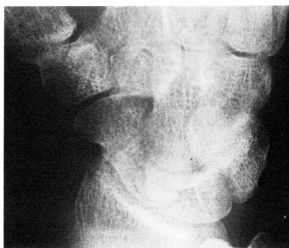

. **Fig. 2.36(a)**   An old fracture of the scaphoid; and **(b)** a recent fracture.

Fig. 2.37   Fracture of the tuberosity of the scaphoid.

Fig. 2.38   Fracture of the waist of the scaphoid.

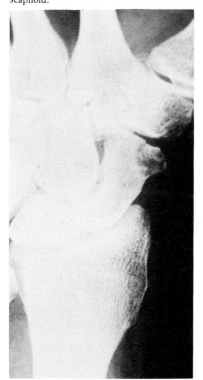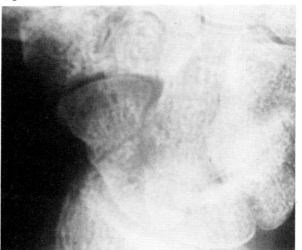

Proximal pole fractures (Fig. 2.39) are treated like the waist fractures, but are often problem fractures due to the small proximal fragment being relatively avascular.

A small avascular fragment (Fig. 2.40) may go on to avascular necrosis and collapse. Once a fragment has been shown to have a poor blood supply (by bone scanning after four weeks) then open reduction internal fixation and bone grafting are advised (Fig. 2.41).

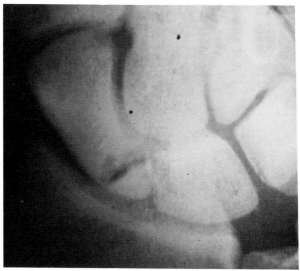

Fig. 2.39   Fracture of the proximal pole of the scaphoid with relative avascularity (increased density).

Fig. 2.40   Bone grafting and internal fixation will be necessary for this avascular proximal pole fracture.

Fig. 2.41   Fixation of a scaphoid fracture with a Herbert screw and bone graft.

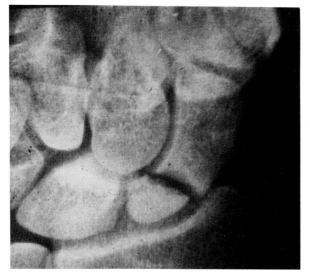

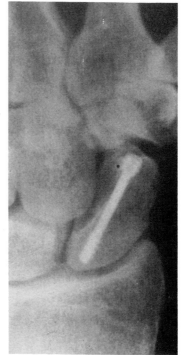

Combined injuries of the scaphoid

Occasionally patients suffer injuries of other bones in combination with the fractured scaphoid bone. A fracture of the distal radius is

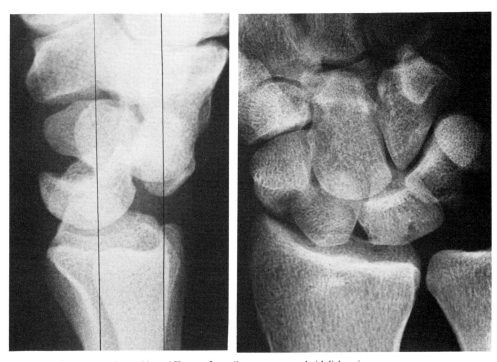

Fig. 2.42 Antero-posterior and lateral X-rays of a perilunate trans-scaphoid dislocation. N.B. The carpus is in two layers.

obvious and presents no problem, however, the X-rays shown in Figure 2.42 do cause problems — study them and see if you can work out what has happened.

Figure 2.42 shows a **perilunate trans-scaphoid dislocation** of the carpal bones, there is a fracture of the scaphoid through its waist the distal half of the scaphoid and the rest of the carpal bones and the hand are dislocated dorsally. *The only bones that are in place are the lunate and the proximal half of the scaphoid.* **This contrasts with dislocations of the lunate** where the lunate is dislocated and the rest of the carpus and hand are in the normal position.

Reduction of the dislocation is not difficult, but the fracture of the scaphoid is unstable and often does not unite — open reduction and fixation of the scaphoid fracture avoids this problem (Fig. 2.43).

Fig. 2.43 X-rays after reduction of the dislocation and internal fixation of the fractured scaphoid.

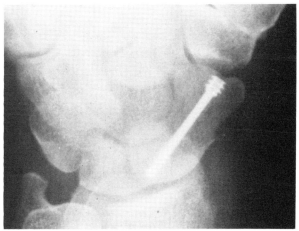

Other carpal bones

There are eight carpal bones and each of them can be fractured, however, the scaphoid bone is by far the most common because it bridges the two rows of the carpus. Most of the other carpal fractures are simple and require immobilization for about four weeks in a short arm plaster and then gentle use for a further month.

Colles' fracture

This is probably the most common fracture that you will have to deal with in casualty. Just for your interest, Abraham Colles was born in Ireland in 1773. Whilst he was at school a flood swept through the local doctor's house carrying away his possessions. One of his anatomy books landed near Colles' house. When Abraham returned it he was given the book to keep. It inspired him.

He obtained his MD in 1797 and then walked from Edinburgh to London (shades of Tom Jones). He was elected President of the Royal College of Surgeons of Ireland at the age of 29 and described radial fractures in 1814 — long before X-rays. He died in 1843. In China it has been known as Wu's fracture for 2000 years.

Colles' fracture is a fracture of the distal end of the radius within 30mm of the wrist joint and commonly, a fracture of the styloid process of the ulna (Fig. 2.44). There is usually dorsal angulation, dorsal and radial rotation and some impaction of the distal fragment on the proximal.

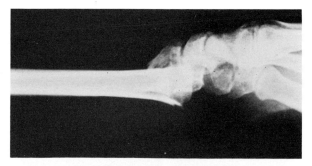

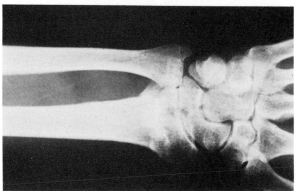

Fig. 2.44   X-rays of a typical Colles' fracture.

The equivalent fracture in a child usually involves the distal radial epiphysis which is similarly displaced but is not impacted.

This fracture gives the classical 'dinner fork' deformity when it is displaced (Fig. 2.45).

Reduction will need to be carried out if:

1. The patient is young and healthy.

2. There is impaction, rotation or angulation, so that on the lateral view the line of the wrist joint is less than vertical.

Conversely, reduction is not necessary in very old and frail people if the deformity including angulation is not gross. It is a

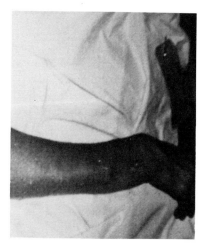

Fig. 2.45   The 'dinner fork' deformity of a Colles' fracture.

general rule that the older and more frail the patient, the more deformity and angulation you can accept.

Reduction and plastering of a Colles' fracture

In line with our previous decision **not to put a full plaster on any recent fracture,** you can plan to put back and side slabs on a Colles' fracture. These can be made from eight thicknesses of plaster of Paris 10cm wide, with one being 25cm long and the other for the radial side being 20cm long. These slabs will be placed on the dorsal and radial aspects of the wrist after the application of some padding — rolled wool, Velband or Webril. The commonest place for a pressure sore after a Colles' fracture is over the ulnar styloid, so be sure that this area is well padded.

Reduction of a Colles' fracture

Reduction is by traction to disimpact the fracture and then by pressure over the displaced distal fragment with your thenar eminence. As you press, you push down in a volar direction and flex the wrist as in Figure 2.46. Now the wrist is semiflexed and in ulnar deviation. **Do not allow any helper to pick up the hand as you apply the plaster as this will redisplace the fracture.**

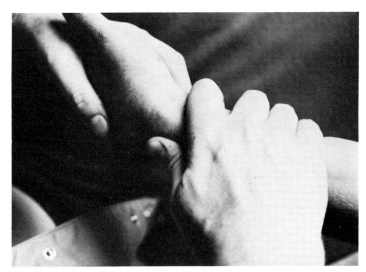

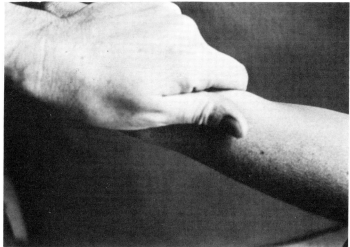

Fig. 2.46(a)   Reduction of a Colles' fracture by traction and dis-impaction; **(b)** followed by direct pressure with the thenar eminence.

Apply the padding (Fig. 2.47), and then the slabs (Fig. 2.48) and mould the plaster as it sets. **You must use a crepe bandage to wrap over the slabs so that the bandage can stretch if swelling occurs** (Fig. 2.49).

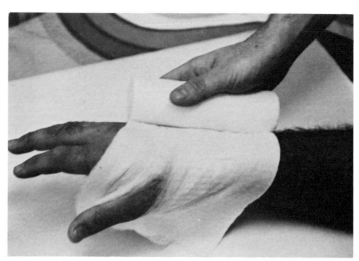

Fig. 2.47   After reduction the arm hangs freely and padding is applied.

The patient should now be instructed to move all the fingers and the thumb regularly and to keep the arm elevated for the next 24 hours. They should then return for a plaster check and the plaster should be trimmed if necessary (especially around the base of the thumb) and a check made on any

Fig. 2.48(a)   The application of back and side slabs; **(b)** bandaged on with a dry crepe bandage and moulding as the plaster sets.

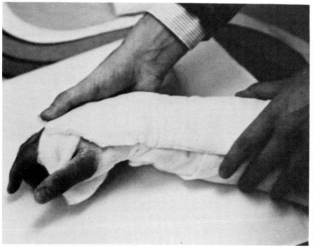
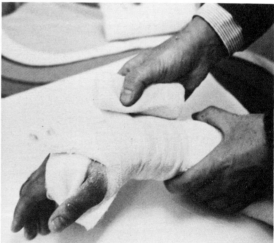

swelling and on the circulation in the hand.

This type of fracture needs to be in plaster for some four to six weeks and then the patient will need another few months of exercising the wrist and hand to regain maximum function. If the patient is a manual worker, he or she will be off work during this time.

Most patients are left with some prominence of the ulnar styloid process due to some impaction of the radius, but they are usually left with an excellent functional result.

Juvenile Colles' fracture

This is the juvenile equivalent of the adult Colles' fracture and involves the distal radial epiphysis (Fig. 2.50). In fact, it is a fracture of the distal end of the radius just proximal to the epiphysis taking a

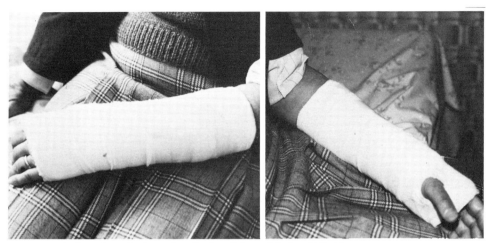

Fig. 2.49 The limb after reduction and application of plaster slabs for a Colles' fracture.

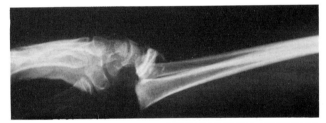

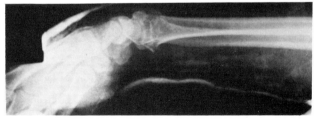

thin slice of bone away with the displaced epiphysis (Fig. 2.51).

The deformity will be similar to that of a Colles' fracture and the treatment will be the same — reduction and plastering in a dorsal and radial slab. Children's fractures often swell a lot, so don't forget to advise the parents that the hand is to be kept elevated and the child is to keep the fingers moving.

Like all children's fractures, this one heals rapidly and needs only three weeks immobilization and a further three weeks of care.

If this fracture has been displaced and then reduced, it could slip from the reduced position, and so needs to be X-rayed after the swelling has gone down (for example, in one week).

Fig. 2.50 Juvenile Colles' fracture with displacement of the distal epiphysis; **(a)** before; and **(b)** after reduction.

Fig. 2.51 The Juvenile Colles' fracture usually has a thin piece of the metaphysis.

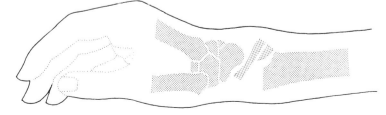

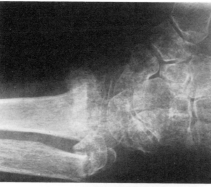

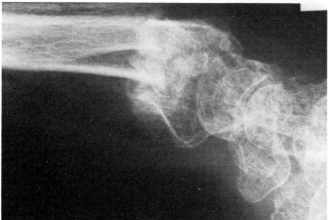

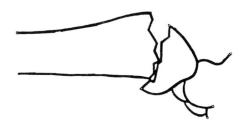

Fig. 2.52   Smith's fracture; **(a)** and **(b)** antero-posterior and lateral X-rays; and **(c)** diagram to show the displacement.

Smith's fracture

This is a reverse Colles' fracture, in which the distal fragment is displaced towards the volar aspect. Smith was also from Dublin and described this fracture in 1847.

In his original article he described it as the frequent result of a fall onto the back of the hand causing a fracture in the distal 3cm of the radius with volar displacement (Fig. 2.52).

Remember that unless you look at the X-rays in the correct way, i.e. with the thumb metacarpal pointing to the floor, you will mistake a Smith's fracture for a Colles' fracture.

All displaced Smith's fractures require reduction and **immobilization in above elbow slabs holding the forearm in full supination** (Fig. 2.53).

Fig. 2.53   Application of backslabs with the arm in full supination for a Smith's fracture.

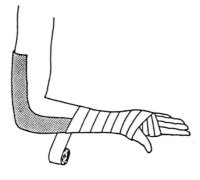

Put your own forearm in full supination with the elbow at 90° (that is with the palm facing upwards) and you can feel how the tightness of the capsule holds the wrist in place. This is the position that you will need to obtain and maintain in order to hold this fracture.

A short arm plaster is unsatisfactory as the forearm can be rotated in pronation and supination (try on your own forearm) **and the fracture will redisplace.**

Reduce the fracture by traction and direct pressure with your thenar eminence over

**the volar aspect of the wrist
(over the distal fragment).** Hold
the forearm in full supination with
pressure over the radial side of the
hand and apply the plaster slabs
over a layer of padding (Fig. 2.53).

**You will need long arm slabs
made up of 12 thicknesses of
10cm wide plaster
approximately 50 cm long.**

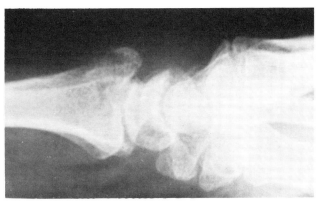

Fig. 2.54   Lateral X-ray of a dorsal type Barton's fracture.

Barton's fracture dislocation

Fig. 2.55   Lateral X-ray of a ventral type Barton's fracture.

In 1838, Barton described a fracture
of the margin of the distal end of the
radius with dislocation of the
carpus. This occurs more often on
the dorsal aspect (Fig. 2.54), but can
occur ventrally (Fig. 2.55). This
fracture of the radius has the dorsal
ligament or the ventral ligament of
the wrist intact, depending on
which way the dislocation occurs.

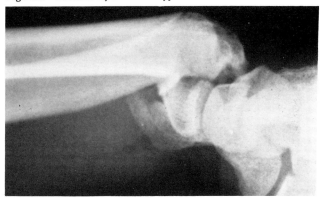

Management

The dislocated carpal bones must be
reduced and held in place, and the
key to this is to reduce and hold the
fracture of the margin of the radius,
and to use the tension of the intact
ligament.

Closed reduction can be done
successfully with traction and direct
pressure over the fragment of radius,
but reduction is often lost as the
swelling subsides and the plaster
loosens. Therefore, during the first
10 days, put the wrist in increased
dorsiflexion (in the ventral type) as
this increases the stability, by
keeping the intact ventral ligament
tense.

Open reduction is often the best
way to handle this difficult fracture
(Fig. 2.56).

N.B. Keep your eyes peeled for
these fractures. They are not
uncommon and are usually labelled
Colles' or Smith's fractures.

Fig. 2.56   Postoperative X-rays after open reduction of a ventral type Barton's fracture.

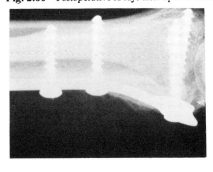
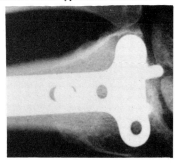

Forearm

Shaft of the radius

Be careful of this innocent looking fracture, unless it is completely undisplaced (Fig. 2.57a). When it is displaced (Fig. 2.57b), be sure the area X-rayed is adequate to assess the problem. There must be another fracture or dislocation in the forearm if there is displacement.

The undisplaced fracture is no problem and only requires immobilization in long arm slabs — these can be tightened with Elastoplast initially and later converted to a full long arm plaster, after the swelling goes down.

A full arm plaster is essential to control pronation and supination.

If there is any displacement then the rectangle (Fig. 2.58) made up by the radius, the ulna, the superior radio-ulnar joint and the inferior radio-ulnar joint must be broken at another point.

This means that you must see the joint above and below the fracture site. If there is displacement at one site in 'the rectangle' then there is another fracture or a dislocation at the proximal or distal radio-ulnar articulation.

A Galeazzi fracture (see next section) is an example of two breaks in the rectangle (Fig. 2.59).

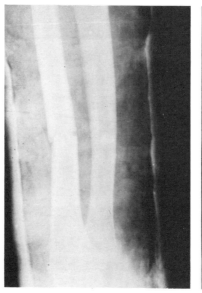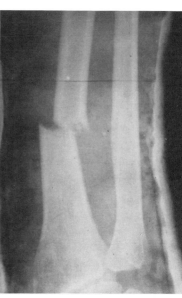

Fig. 2.57(a)   Undisplaced; and **(b)** displaced fractures of the shaft of the radius in plaster.

Fig. 2.58   The rectangle concept – radius (R), wrist joint (W), ulna (U) and elbow joint (E).

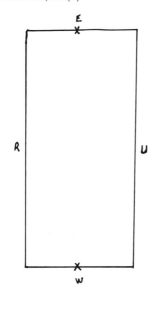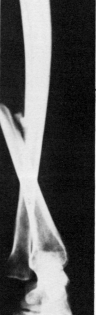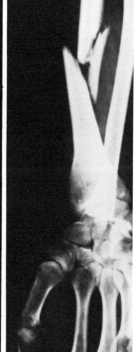

Fig. 2.59   Galeazzi's fracture.

Galeazzi's fracture

Riccardo Galeazzi was an Italian 20th century surgeon who came from Milan, the same place as Monteggia. Between them they described fractures of the lower and upper forearm.

Galeazzi lived from 1866 to 1952 and was director of an orthopaedic clinic for 35 years. He wrote on many subjects and reviewed 12 000 cases of congenital dislocation of the hip. His article on this fracture was written in 1934.

A Galeazzi fracture is a fracture of the radius, usually at the junction of the middle and distal thirds, with a dislocation of the ulna at the distal radio-ulnar joint (Figs. 2.60). It is not an uncommon injury — about 6 per cent of all forearm fractures.

Galeazzi advocated closed reduction by 'energetic traction' on the thumb with the hand in supination and then radial deviation to reduce the dislocated 'ulnar head'. A long arm plaster for ten weeks was advocated. Unfortunately the results of this closed treatment are not good, as the dislocation can recur and since the fracture is often slow to unite, it is difficult to hold in position. The unstable nature of the fracture is well shown in Figure 2.61.

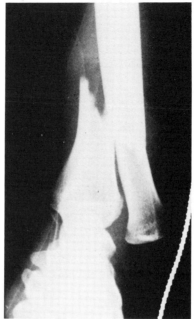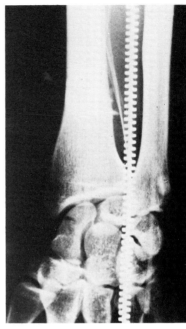

Fig. 2.60   Lateral and antero-posterior X-rays of a Galeazzi fracture.

Fig. 2.61   Galeazzi's fracture – note the distal ulna dislocation.

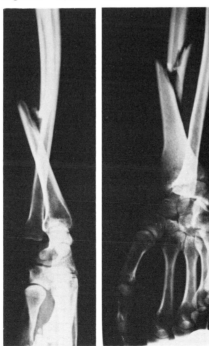

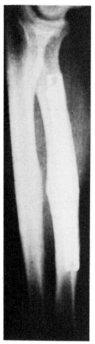
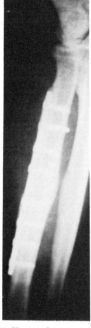

Fig. 2.62 Postoperative X-rays of a Galeazzi fracture, after three months.

Operative treatment usually includes compression plating of the fracture of the radius (Fig. 2.62), and occasionally a threaded pin is placed temporarily across the lower radio-ulnar joint.

Shaft of the ulna

Isolated fractures of the shaft of the ulna are fairly common and are usually the result of direct trauma.

Figure 2.63 shows the X-rays of a patient who was struck by a golf ball. Similar injuries can occur when you put your arm up to protect your face and your attacker hits your ulna with a heavy object such as a stick or a hammer.

Initially, this fracture will need to be treated in long arm slabs. These can be tightened with Elastoplast

Fig. 2.63 Fracture of the shaft of the ulna from a direct blow.

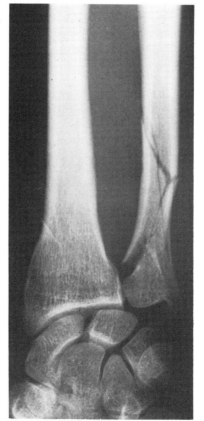

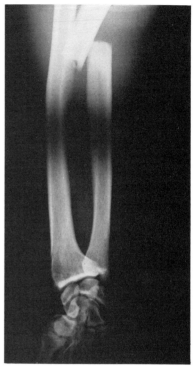

Fig. 2.64 Fracture of the shaft of the ulna with displacement . . . beware.

(see *Circulatory problems*, Ch. 1) or replaced with a long arm plaster when the swelling has gone down. Immobilization will need to be continued for six to eight weeks.

It is important to realise that the rectangle concept (see Fig. 2.58) applies to the ulna as well as the radius.

Remember that if there is a displaced fracture of the ulna (Fig. 2.64), there must be another fracture present or a dislocation of the superior or inferior radio-ulnar joints.

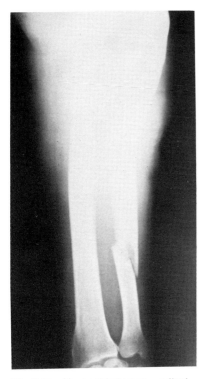

Fig. 2.65 Monteggia's fracture − a distal fracture of the ulna. Elbow not seen.

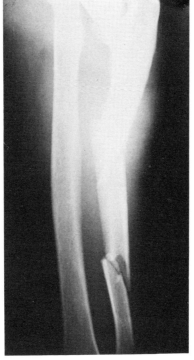

Fig. 2.66 Monteggia's fracture with, the often missed, dislocation of the head of the radius.

Monteggia's fracture dislocation

Giovanni Battista Monteggia (1762-1815) was a surgical pathologist who later became professor of surgery at Milan. He described his fracture in the same year as Colles described his more famous fracture of the wrist (1814). In fact Monteggia described how he failed to diagnose the fracture and failed to treat the lesion, but he did describe the fracture dislocation.

Monteggia's fracture is a fracture of the proximal third of the ulna with a dislocation of the head of the radius (Figs. 2.67a and b). It occurs in both children and in adults, and whilst the fracture of the ulna is obvious, **the lesion that is missed is the dislocation of the head of the radius.**

A Monteggia fracture, i.e. a fracture of the ulna shaft usually in the upper third and a dislocation of the head of the radius (Figs. 2.65 and 2.66), is an example of two breaks in the rectangle (see Fig. 2.58).

Fig. 2.67 The common ventral type of Monteggia's fracture.

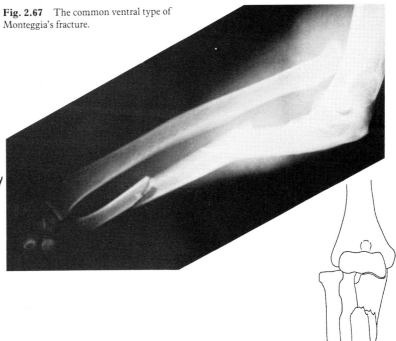

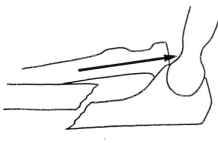

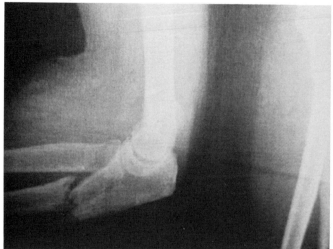

Fig. 2.68   The dorsal type of Monteggia's fracture.

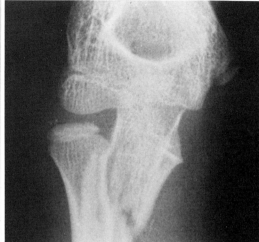

Fig. 2.69   The rare lateral type of Monteggia's fracture.

There are three types of Monteggia fracture depending on the direction of the deformity of the ulna and dislocation of the radial head. The ventral type (Figs. 2.67a and b) is the most common (85 per cent), followed by the dorsal (10 per cent) (Fig. 2.68) and the lateral (Fig. 2.69).

In the lateral and in the antero-posterior view, the head of the radius should line up with the middle of the capitellum — failure to reduce this dislocation will prevent normal elbow movement, particularly in rotation of the forearm (pronation and supination).

Management

Monteggia's fracture dislocation requires reduction of both the fracture and the dislocation (Fig. 2.70).

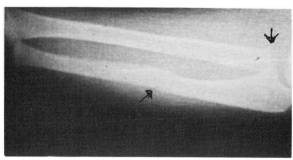

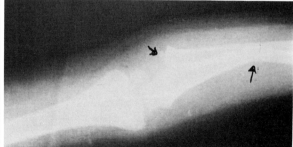

Fig. 2.70   Pressure points used in reduction of a Monteggia fracture.

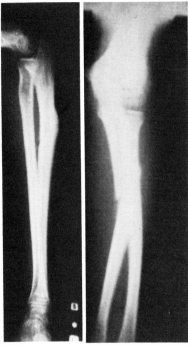

Fig. 2.71   Post reduction X-rays of a Monteggia fracture – both components are well reduced.

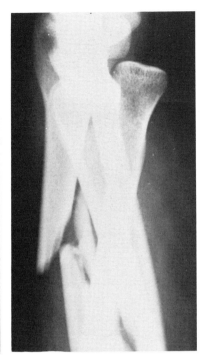

Fig. 2.72   Unstable Monteggia fracture needing internal fixation.

Fig. 2.73   Open reduction and compression plating of the Monteggia fracture shown in Figure 2.72.

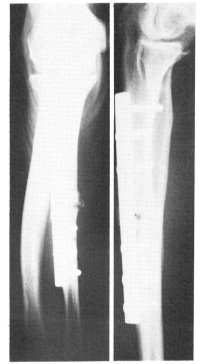

In children, closed reduction by traction and direct pressure over the radial head usually works well (Fig. 2.71).

Immobilize the child in long arm slabs (front and back) and check the reduction on X-ray. A further check will be necessary in one week when the plaster can be tightened or completed.

In adults, the lesion is often much more unstable (Fig. 2.72) and although reduction is possible (as above) the fracture and the dislocation tend to slip. Open reduction and compression plating of the fractured ulna and closed reduction of the dislocated radial head is the treatment of choice (Fig. 2.73). Whilst awaiting operation the patient should be immobilized in a long (arm), well padded backslab.

Both bones of the forearm

Adult

Unless this fracture is undisplaced or can be reduced and maintained in nearly perfect position (Fig. 2.74), problems will arise in that not only does the forearm need to be straight with the radius and ulna in correct alignment, but these two forearm bones need to remain parallel if the radius is to rotate on the ulna (Fig. 2.75).

Open reduction and internal fixation will be necessary for all displaced fractures of the forearm in adults (Fig. 2.76).

This is not an urgent procedure, unless the circulation is in doubt or the fracture is compound. While waiting for the operation, a long arm plaster should be applied **over suitable padding** and is immediately **split down to the skin** (Fig. 2.77), **or alternately long arm slabs are applied over suitable padding.**

Analgesics, elevation, and a circulation check will be necessary.

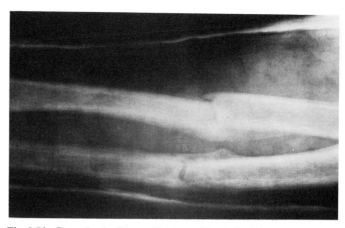

Fig. 2.74   Post reduction X-rays of fractures of the shafts of the radius and ulna in good position.

Fig. 2.75   Post reduction X-rays of radius and ulna – they are parallel.

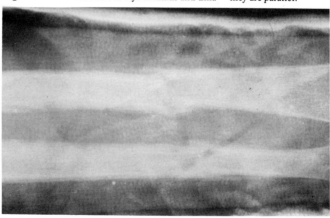

Fig. 2.76   Open reduction of fractures of the shafts of the radius and ulna with compression plates: **(a)** before; and **(b)** after.

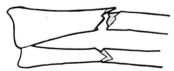

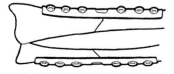

Fig. 2.77   A long arm plaster in mid position between pronation and supination – split along the dotted line to allow for swelling.

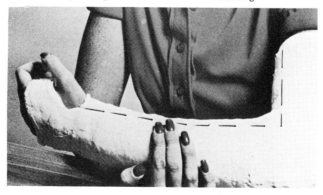

Children — distal end

A greenstick or an undisplaced fracture (Fig. 2.78) can be put in dorsal and radial short arm slabs over a layer of padding.

When there is angulation (Fig. 2.79) this will need to be reduced and dorsal and radial short arm plaster slabs will be necessary.

However, this fracture is commonly displaced, as shown in Fig. 2.80, and can be difficult to reduce.

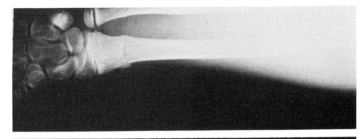

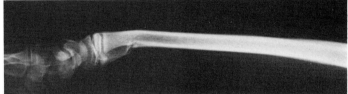

Fig. 2.78   Greenstick fracture of the distal third of the radius and ulna.

Fig. 2.79   Fractures of distal thirds of the radius and ulna with gross angulation.

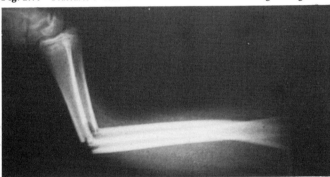

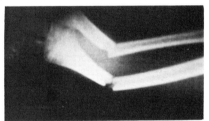

Fig. 2.80   X-rays of fractures of the distal thirds of the radius and ulna with full width displacement dorsally.

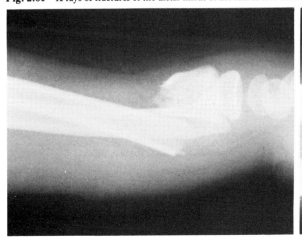

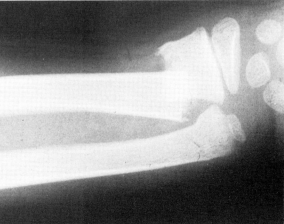

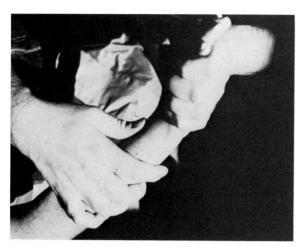

Fig. 2.81 Technique of disimpaction of the fractures shown in Figure 2.80.

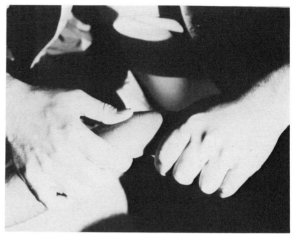

Fig. 2.82 Technique of reduction after disimpaction.

Where the fracture is displaced a reduction under a general anaesthetic will often be necessary. Figures 2.81 and 2.82 show how the fracture needs to be handled. In order to reduce this fracture, you have to increase the deformity (Fig. 2.81) and push the base of the fracture (the proximal part of the distal fragment) into place (Fig. 2.82) and then correct the angulation. Finally, immobilize the arm in long arm plaster slabs (Fig. 2.83) and the plaster will need to be kept on for about four weeks. **Please note that this fracture can displace easily (Fig. 2.84) and a check X-ray should be done during the reduction and again at one week.** At this stage, the plaster can be tightened or completed — or if the fracture has slipped, a further reduction can be carried out (Fig. 2.85).

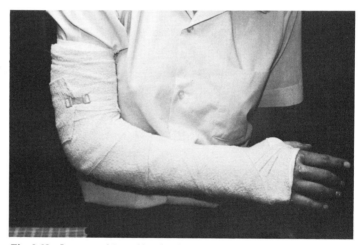

Fig. 2.83 Long arm slabs and bandage in a child.

Fig. 2.84 This fracture is not reduced well enough.

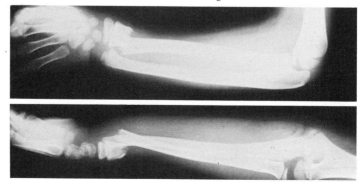

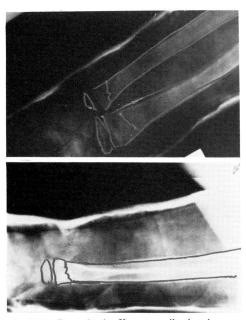

Fig. 2.85 Post reduction X-rays − well reduced.

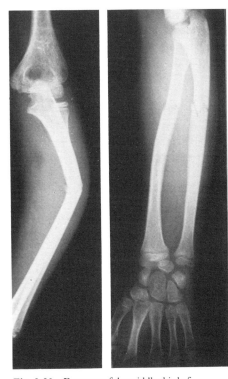

Fig. 2.86 Fractures of the middle third of the radius and ulna with gross angulation.

Fig. 2.87 X-rays showing good reduction of the fracture shown in Figure 2.86.

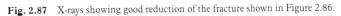

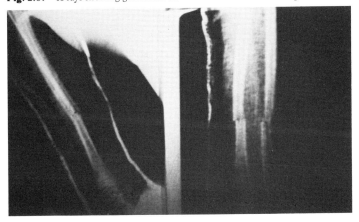

Children — middle third

This fracture can also be difficult to reduce and to hold, but because we can reduce the fracture repeatedly if necessary and nature will remould some angulation and displacement, we can accept a reduction that would not be acceptable in an adult.

Reduction. An angulated fracture (Fig. 2.86) is reduced by direct pressure and a forceful push on the distal radius and ulna. The arm is then immobilized in long arm plaster slabs and X-rayed (Fig. 2.87) to check the reduction.

A displaced fracture of this type is more difficult and needs traction to increase the deformity, then the bone ends must be hooked together, before pressing the bones into alignment. I find it best to mould the fracture and hook the bones onto each other, whilst one helper holds down the arm just above the elbow and another exerts strong traction vertically, such that the fingertips point to the ceiling and the radius and ulna are in the midposition as far as pronation and supination are concerned.

How much deformity and angulation can be accepted?

This depends on two factors:

1. The age of the child. The younger the child the more angulation can be accepted and, the quicker remodelling will take place to return the bone to normal. At birth, an angulation of 90° will correct itself and at the age of ten, about 20° angulation will remodel completely within twelve months.

2. The closer the deformity is to the epiphysis, the greater the correction and the quicker it will occur. In other words, a fracture at the distal end of the bone will correct more quickly and completely than a fracture in the middle of the bone.

If you warn parents that there will be a bump or angulation early in the treatment, they will then accept it. However, if you do not warn them and they see it after you take the plaster off, they will tend not to believe you when you advise that correction will occur in the next few months.

Elbow fractures in children

General

As we can see from the X-rays and diagrams below there are problems for the casualty officer in recognising fractures in this area and distinguishing them from epiphyseal lines.

Remember:

1. You can and should X-ray the other elbow and compare them.

2. Fracture lines are thin and jagged, whereas epiphyseal lines are wide and smooth.

3. Fractures are very tender and painful to pressure.

The epiphyses around the elbow are shown in Figure 2.88.

Medial and lateral humeral condyles

These fractures are relatively common and are important in that they often involve the epiphyses and are intra-articular. Failure to manage this fracture properly when displaced (Fig. 2.89) will lead to an ugly deformity (Fig. 2.90). When they are undisplaced, the fracture requires only immobilization in a backslab and a sling for three weeks. **When there is displacement of the fragment open reduction and fixation by K-wires is necessary** (Fig. 2.91).

Apply a backslab to control pain while the patient is awaiting operation.

Fig. 2.88   Epiphyses around the elbow joint. N.B. They are not fractures.

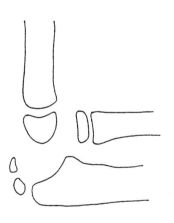

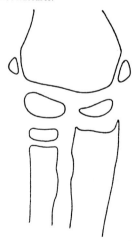

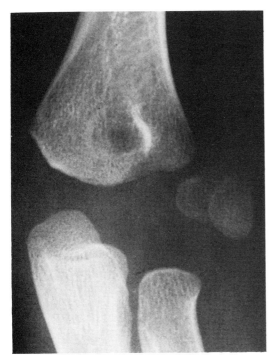

Fig. 2.89 Displaced fracture of the lateral condyle of the humerus.

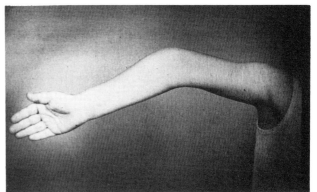

Fig. 2.90 Ugly deformity from a malunited fracture of the medial condyle.

Fig. 2.91 Excellent reduction and K-wire fixation of a fracture of the lateral condyle of the humerus.

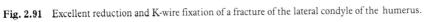

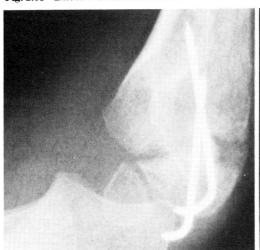

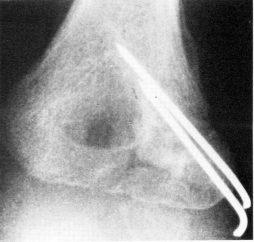

Medial epicondyle of the humerus

Beware of this trap. The epiphysis of the medial epicondyle appears at the age of five and thereafter must always be seen on X-rays of the elbow, and **be seen to be in place.** If it is displaced it will need to be openly reduced and fixed with K-wires, as the common flexor origin will keep it in the displaced position. **Both this fracture and fractures of the condyles rotate when they displace and cannot be held reduced by closed means.**

Figures 2.92a, b, c and d show the medial epicondyle displaced and in the joint. This probably occurs when the joint momentarily dislocates and then comes back into place, trapping the medial epicondyle. Even when the joint is dislocated (Figs. 2.92c, d and e) you should look for the epicondyle and be aware that during reduction it may jam in the joint.

Apply a padded backslab for the patient's comfort whilst awaiting operation.

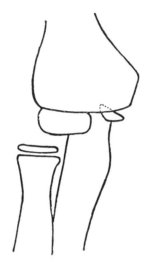

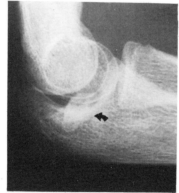

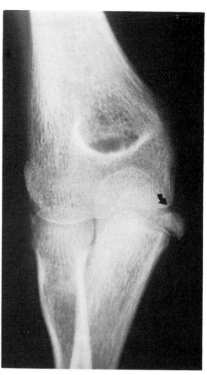

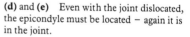

Fig. 2.92(a), (b) and **(c)**   The disappearing medial epicondyle. Where is it? The arrows shows it in the joint.

(d) and **(e)**   Even with the joint dislocated, the epicondyle must be located – again it is in the joint.

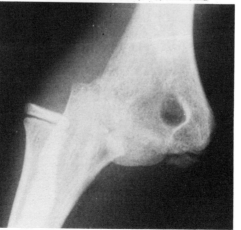

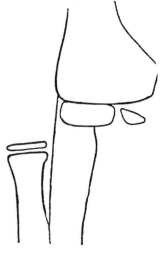

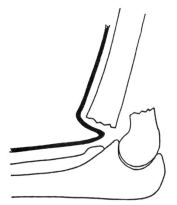

Fig. 2.93 Arterial kinking and spasm is a common cause of problems.

Supracondylar fractures of the humerus

This fracture has a bad reputation, but it is my view that only a very small number of cases need be left with any residual problems provided care, diligence and skill are exercised.

The possible residual problems must be understood in order to prevent their occurrence. They are:

1. Vascular impairment (Fig. 2.93) due to arterial damage or arterial compression by too much flexion, or a full plaster. This can cause permanent damage to muscles and nerves in the forearm, and is known as Volkmann's ischaemic contracture (Fig. 2.94).

2. Deformity at the elbow joint and loss of or increased carrying angle of the arm, due to acceptance of varus or valgus deformity. Loss of flexion may be due to acceptance of posterior angulation. Rotatory deformity is also a type of malposition.

3. Marked residual stiffness is usually due to someone passively manipulating the elbow (rather than actively exercising) or too many attempts at reduction. A full range of movements (Figs. 2.95a and b) is possible in most cases.

Fig. 2.94 Volkmann's ischaemia can cause serious muscle and nerve damage in the forearm and hand.

Fig. 2.95 A full range of movement should return after a supracondylar fracture.

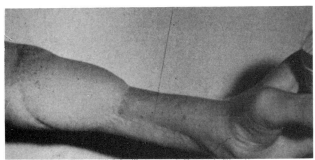

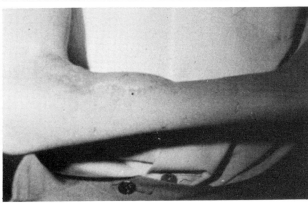

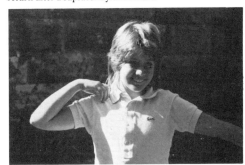

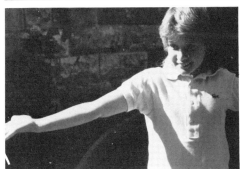

Undisplaced supracondylar fractures

This fracture (Figs. 2.96a and b) requires immobilization in a simple backslab with the elbow at ninety degrees — after a generous layer of padding has been applied. If you simply put the arm in an inside collar and cuff you are not really immobilizing the fracture very well, and the child will continue to cry all night.

The angry parents will descend on you the next morning when the child is brought back for the routine follow-up check because the child will have had unnecessary pain.

This fracture requires three weeks immobilization and then **active** exercises with care for a further period of three weeks. Full return of function can be anticipated. The child should be kept away from sport and vigorous activity for six to eight weeks. Keep the arm inside the clothes whilst it is being immobilized.

Displaced supracondylar fractures

Please check the circulation in the hand on arrival in casualty and if there is no circulation arrange immediate reduction as this is a surgical emergency. Do not wait for X-rays — even a partial reduction produced by traction and slight flexion will

Fig. 2.96   Lateral and antero-posterior X-rays of an undisplaced supracondylar fracture.

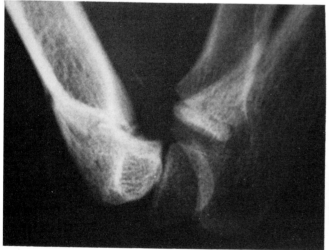
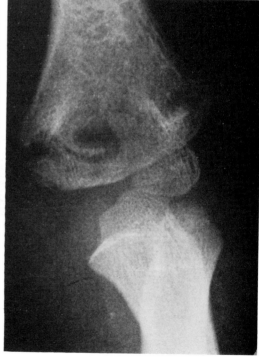

usually free the artery from pressure and restore the circulation (Fig. 2.97).

If the circulation is satisfactory, apply a simple splint and arrange for the arm to be X-rayed — **keep a watch on the circulation.**

Let us look at the X-rays of the displaced supracondylar fractures (Fig. 2.98a and b) and work out our plan of reduction.

There are three types of problem:

1. The supracondylar fracture with anterior displacement.

2. The supracondylar fracture with posterior and medial displacement.

3. The supracondylar fracture with posterior and lateral displacement.

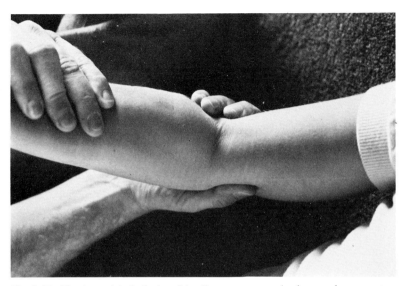

Fig. 2.97   Traction and slight flexion of the elbow to ease acute circulatory embarrassment in casualty.

Fig. 2.98(a) and **(b)**   A-P and Lateral X-ray of a displaced supracondylar fracture of the humerus.

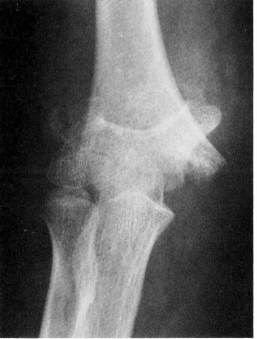
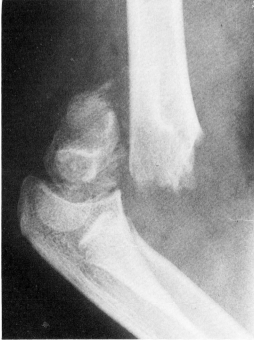

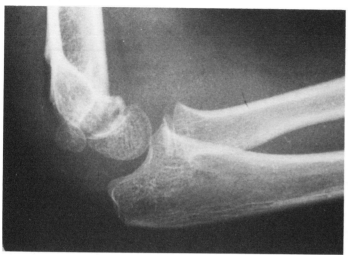
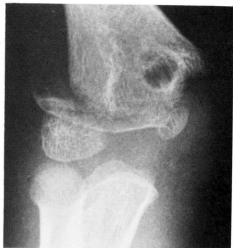

Fig. 2.99   Lateral and antero-posterior X-rays of the rare supracondylar fracture of the humerus with anterior and lateral displacement.

1. *The supracondylar fracture with anterior displacement of the distal fragment (Figs. 2.99a and b)*

A rare problem, and one that I mention first so that you will keep it in mind. It is uncommon (only 4 per cent of supracondylar fractures are of this type). Please look at the X-rays and **see if the displaced distal fragment is anterior or posterior.**

   This fracture requires reduction by pressure in a posterior direction over the distal fragment. If it is stable in a semi-flexed position then it should be maintained this way, but usually it is only stable in extension. Do not keep the arm fully extended for more than ten days. At the end of this time the fracture will be sticky and the elbow can be flexed gently under analgesia and maintained in this position for a further ten days. **Remember if your elbow is stiff in extension your hand cannot reach your mouth or your pocket.**

2. *The supracondylar fracture with posterior and medial displacement of the distal fragment (Figs. 2.100a and b)*

This is the most common supracondylar fracture. Here the periosteal hinge is intact on the medial side and the fracture can be

Fig. 2.100(a) and **(b)**   Lateral and antero-posterior X-rays of a supracondylar fracture of the humerus with posterior and medial displacement.

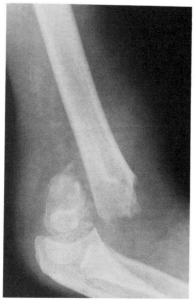
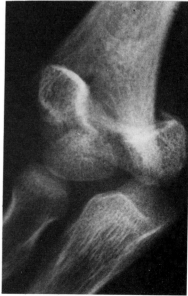

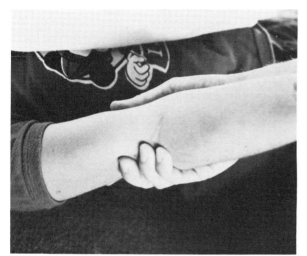

Fig. 2.101 Traction and realignment of the supracondylar fracture.

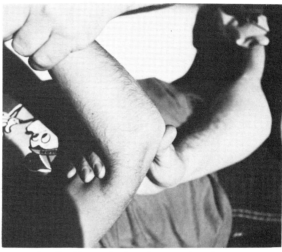

Fig. 2.102 Pushing on the distal fragment through the olecranon with your thumb.

reduced and held as follows:

1. Traction on the hand with the child under a relaxant general anaesthetic (Fig. 2.101).

2. Correction of the medial displacement and rotation of the distal fragment, so that the distal fragment lies in alignment with the shaft of the humerus but is posterior to it (Fig. 2.101).

3. Traction on the forearm, and direct thumb pressure over the olecranon as the elbow is flexed. The distal fragment should then slide forward in place (Fig. 2.102). Check the radial pulse (Fig. 2.103) as you flex the elbow.

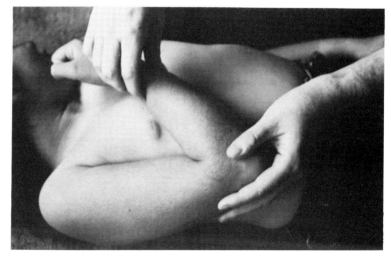

Fig. 2.103 Check the radial pulse as you decide on how much flexion.

4. The medial hinge is now closed by pronating the forearm so that the hand faces away from the child's body and toward the ceiling (Figs. 2.104a and b).

Having reduced the fracture and confirmed this on X-ray, how will we immbolize the arm?

Either

In an inside collar and cuff next to the skin and under all clothes with the knots taped — so that well meaning but misguided people cannot undo the arm and exercise it.

Or

In a backslab (most people will not touch this and so your well meaning but interfering parent (or friend) will not alter your reduced position).

Do not under ANY CIRCUMSTANCES put a full plaster on the arm!

The child remains in hospital and careful observation of the circulation in the hand is carried out, because we have both reduced the fracture and flexed the elbow, it only takes a little swelling in the closed space to embarrass the circulation (Fig. 2.105).

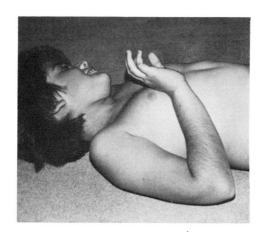

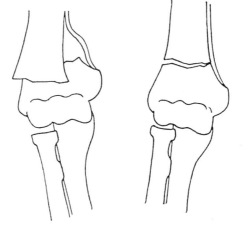
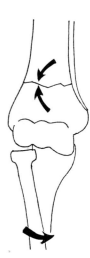

Fig. 2.104(a)   Close the medial hinge by pronating the forearm.
(b) How it works in theory.

Fig. 2.105(a)   The fractured elbow is like a balloon; and **(b)** when you bend it, you can kink and compress the artery.

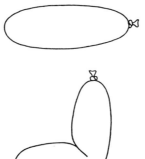

The arm should lie across the child's chest and is thus uppermost so that the circulation can be checked easily (Fig. 2.106) and the child must be encouraged to move the fingers. If the fingers go blue, cold, or there is loss of sensation and undue pain, then an urgent circulation problem exists and must be corrected by undoing the degree of flexion.

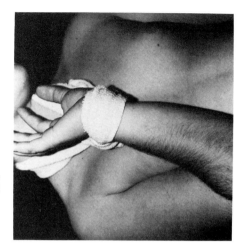

Fig. 2.106 The position of immobilization of the supracondylar fracture of the humerus with medial displacement after reduction.

3. *The supracondylar fracture with posterior and lateral displacement (Figs. 2.107a and b)*

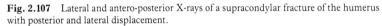

Fig. 2.107 Lateral and antero-posterior X-rays of a supracondylar fracture of the humerus with posterior and lateral displacement.

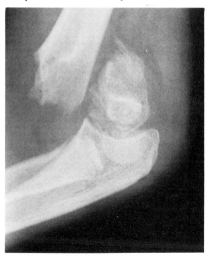
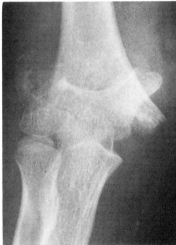

This is the second most common variety of this fracture. Here the periosteal hinge is on the lateral side and the fracture can be reduced and held as follows:

1. Traction on the hand with the child under a relaxant general anaesthetic (Fig. 2.108).

2. Correction of the lateral displacement and rotation of the distal fragment, so that the distal fragment lies in alignment with the shaft of the humerus but is posterior to it (Fig. 2.108).

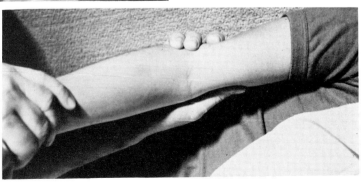

Fig. 2.108 Traction and correction of the alignment of the humerus.

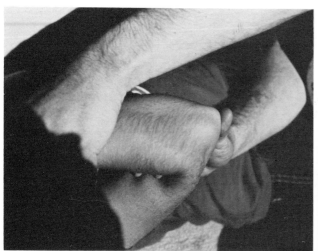

Fig. 2.109 Correction of the posterior displacement by thumb pressure through the olecranon.

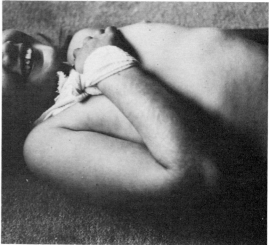

Fig. 2.110 Closure of the lateral hinge of periosterum and the position of immobilization.

3. Traction on the forearm and direct pressure by your thumb over the olecranon as the elbow is flexed. The distal fragment should then slide forward in place (Fig. 2.109).

4. The lateral hinge is now closed by supinating the forearm so that the hand faces toward the child's body and towards the floor (Fig. 2.110).

Immobilization is the same as for the medial displacement type of fracture and is detailed above.

Ask yourself two questions during reduction:

1. **Is reduction satisfactory? How much displacement and angulation can I accept?**

The answer is that you cannot accept ANY angulation or rotation (Fig. 2.111) and there should be as little displacement as possible — perfect reduction gives better stability and less chance of

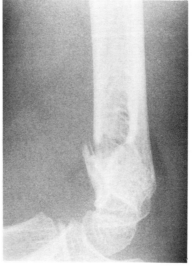
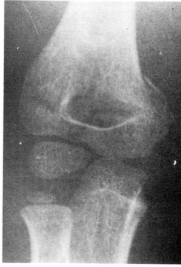

Fig. 2.111 Lateral and antero-posterior X-rays of a well reduced supracondylar fracture.

displacement during the next few days. However, displacement without angulation and rotation is acceptable. Remoulding during growth will correct any displacement that was accepted, but it will not correct angulation or rotation.

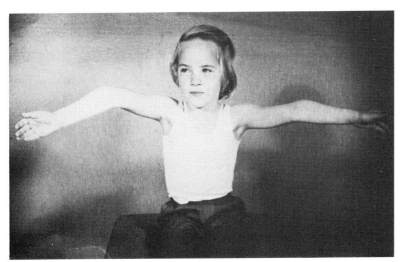

Fig. 2.112 Cubitus varus deformity from a malunion of a supracondylar fracture.

Fig. 2.113 Unsatisfactory position of a supracondylar fracture.

Fig. 2.114 Unsatisfactory position of a supracondylar fracture.

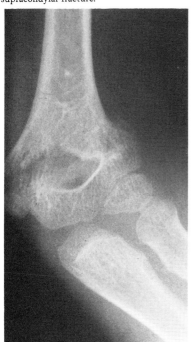

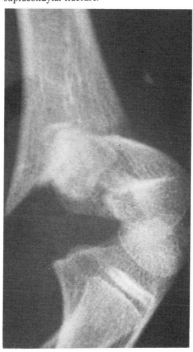

Cubitus varus (Fig. 2.112) and cubitus valgus are very ugly deformities and are always a result of malunion due to a poor original position after reduction (Figs. 2.113 and 2.114) or subsequent slipping of the reduction.

2. **How much can I flex the elbow and improve the stability, without compromising the circulation?**

The answer of course depends on the amount of swelling present. I suggest that you flex the elbow to the point where the pulse disappears, which is obviously too far, and then lessen the flexion by 20°. If the circulation is now clearly adequate, then this is the position of immobilization.

Flex it more for stability — flex it less for circulation.

Open reduction of this fracture is rarely required (Fig. 2.115) but is necessary if exploration of the artery is carried out. Some surgeons will carry out percutaneous pinning (Fig. 2.116) in unstable fractures.

Post reduction regime. **The patient will require hourly checking of the pulse and capillary return. If there is a problem, then flexion needs to be undone until the circulation is no longer in doubt, even if it means the reduction is lost.** *If reduction is lost re-reduce when the swelling has gone down, i.e. in two or three days.*

A check X-ray needs to be done 24-48 hours after the reduction. If this is satisfactory, the circulation is good and the swelling is not a problem, the child can go home. One week later the reduction is checked on X-ray — *re-reduce if necessary.*

It is essential that the parents understand the importance of the fracture being held in place **by the elbow remaining flexed and under the clothes (Fig. 2.117).**

This fracture requires three weeks immobilization and then active exercises *not passive exercises.* If reduction has been good and the fracture remains in a good position, then a good result will ensue but, depending a little on the age of the child, it may take as long as one year for a full range of movement to return.

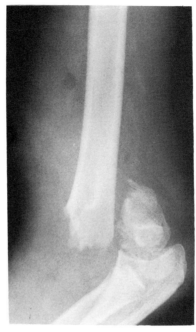

Fig. 2.115   Lateral X-ray of a supracondylar fracture that was associated with damage to the brachial artery.

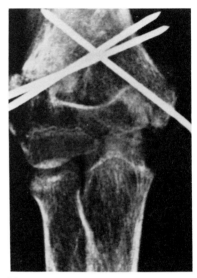

Fig. 2.116   Heavy K-wires used to transfix the fracture shown in Figure 2.115.

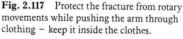

Fig. 2.117   Protect the fracture from rotary movements while pushing the arm through clothing – keep it inside the clothes.

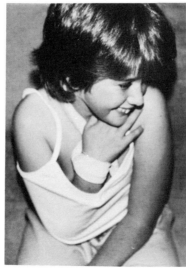

What do you do if the elbow and hand are so grossly swollen that you are unable to flex the elbow?

When there is so much swelling, it is impossible to attempt reduction until the swelling goes down a little. In these circumstances, I suggest that the elbow be immobilized by overhead traction (Fig. 2.118). This requires the insertion of a screw in the ulna distal to the proximal epiphysis and the suspension of the arm in an 'overhead' position.

Skin traction (Fig. 2.119) or Dunlop's traction in a modified Thomas splint can be used but is harder to control and is not as comfortable for the child.

Neck of the radius

This is a common fracture and you will need to look carefully at the X-rays to assess the degree of angulation, since this determines the treatment. There are three types of problem (Fig. 2.120):

1. Undisplaced, or angulated up to 30 degrees (Fig. 2.120A, B).

2. Angulated more than 30 degrees (Fig. 2.120C).

3. Completely displaced and/or associated with a displaced fracture of the proximal ulna (Fig. 2.120D).

Assessment of X-rays

Hold the X-ray so that the shaft of the radius and ulna are vertical. You can then see how far the head of the radius is tilted. It should sit like a

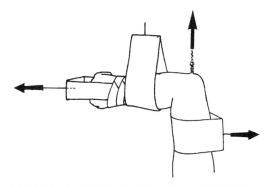

Fig. 2.118   Overhead traction through a screw in the ulna.

Fig. 2.119   Skin traction to maintain alignment.

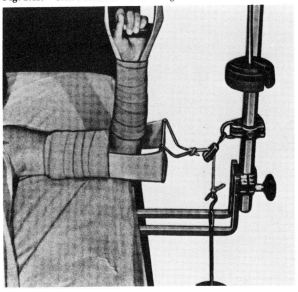

Fig. 2.120   Types of fractures of the neck of the radius.

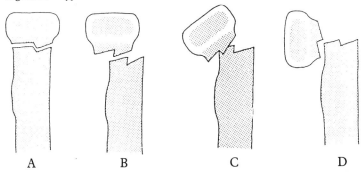

A   B   C   D

cap on a bottle and the plane of the head of the radius should be at right angles to the shaft of the radius.

1. *No displacement or less than 30 degrees angulation (Fig. 2.121)*

This fracture (Fig. 2.122) will recover without any help from the treating doctor, and you can be sure that full function will return. However, it is quite painful for the child and warrants a long arm backslab to immobilize the elbow and prevent pronation and supination. A backslab is preferable to an inside collar and cuff because if the arm is bumped, the plaster will protect the fracture and prevent pain.

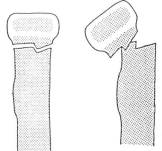

Fig. 2.121   Undisplaced fractures or those with less than 30 per cent angulation.

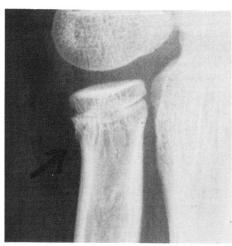

Fig. 2.122   Antero-posterior X-ray of a fracture of the neck of the radius with a small degree of angulation.

Fig. 2.123   Antero-posterior X-ray of a more than 30 per cent angulation.

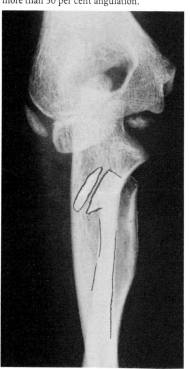

2. *Angulation of more than 30 degrees.*

This will require reduction (Fig. 2.123) as nature cannot overcome this degree of deformity.

Reduction will need to be under general anaesthesia.

Put a varus strain on the elbow, i.e. try and open up the lateral side and push against the head of the radius postero-medially whilst rotating the forearm (Fig. 2.124).

Fig. 2.124   Technique of reduction of the fracture shown in Figure 2.123.

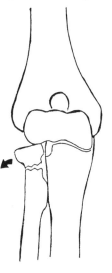
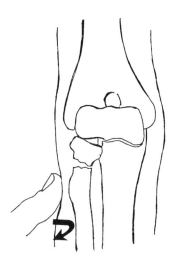

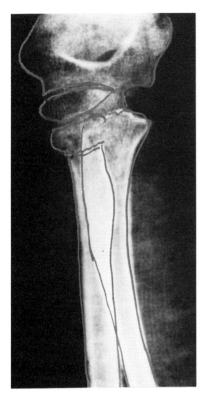

Fig. 2.125 Post reduction X-ray of Figure 2.123.

Check the reduction on X-ray:

a. If successful (Fig. 2.125), apply a long arm backslab over padding.

b. If unsuccessful, then repeat the manoeuvre using more traction on the arm. If again unsuccessful then open reduction will be necessary.

3. *Irreducible angulation over 30 degrees and where there is also a displaced fracture of the ulna which cannot be reduced.*

This means that open operation is required. Even in cases where the head of the radius is right off there is almost always a periosteal bridge which will ensure the survival of the head — **the head is not excised and is pushed back into place.** Removal of the head will lead to a cubitus valgus deformity and late development of an ulnar nerve palsy as the carrying angle of the elbow increases with growth.

Please warn the child's parents,

that with any displaced fracture of the neck of the radius it will take a long time for rotation to return, but the end result will be good. Open reduction can lead to some loss of rotation and as the results of open reduction are not as good as closed reduction, try hard to reduce it by closed means.

Olecranon

Isolated fractures of the olecranon are rare in children. However, fractures with separation may occur, particularly in open fractures due to direct trauma (Figs. 2.126a and b).

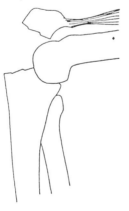
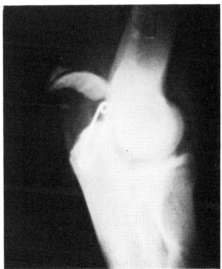

Fig. 2.126 Fracture of the olecranon showing the displacement due to the pull of the triceps.

They require reduction and usually
fixation by the tension band method
(Fig. 2.127).

**Beware of the trap of the
unreduced dislocation of the
head of the radius associated
with a fracture of the olecranon
or even more commonly with a
more distal ulna fracture in the
middle thirds of the bone.
Always check and recheck to
see that the radial head is not
too far anterior in the lateral
view.**

(This is a Monteggia type fracture.)
The trap is that the eyes are
attracted to the obvious fracture of
the ulna and the dislocation of the
radial head is missed twice — firstly,
on the initial X-rays and secondly,
and more importantly on **the post
reduction X-rays (Figs. 2.128a
and b).**

In the case of an anterior
dislocation of the radial head,
reduction will need to be maintained
with the elbow well flexed.

(See the previous section on
**Monteggia's fracture of the
forearm.)**

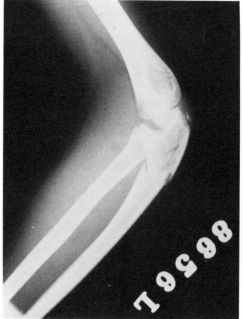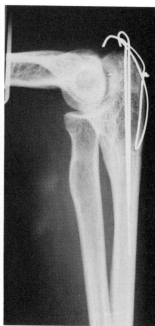

Fig. 2.127   Lateral X-rays of a fracture of the olecranon treated by tension band wiring.

Fig. 2.128   Lateral and antero-posterior X-rays of elbows with the radius still dislocated.

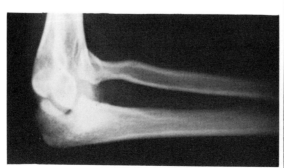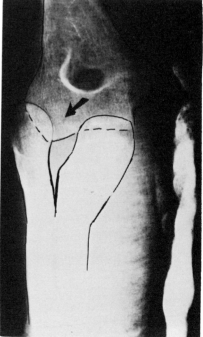

Elbow fractures in adults

Head of the radius

This is a relatively common fracture (Fig. 2.129) and may or may not be a problem depending on the amount of damage that has occurred and the success of our efforts to repair them. After all, it is an intra-articular fracture and therefore there will be equivalent damage to the capitellum whenever there is extensive damage to the head of the radius. Figure 2.129 shows some of the patterns of fracture.

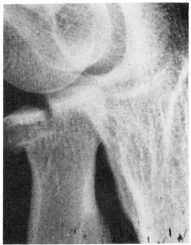
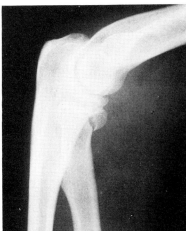
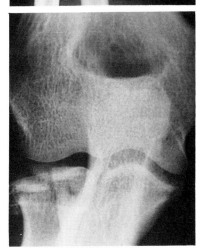

Fig. 2.129 Some X-rays of differing fractures of the head of the radius.

Undisplaced fractures of the radial head

This fracture (Fig. 2.130) requires immobilization in a plaster backslab for three weeks and then active exercises. They require six weeks away from sport.

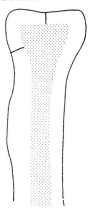

Fig. 2.130 Undisplaced crack fracture of the head of the radius.

Displaced and comminuted fractures

Displaced fractures require open reduction and internal fixation (Fig. 2.131). They must be perfectly reduced (Fig. 2.132) and fixed, if full function is to be obtained.

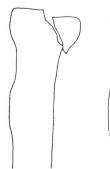
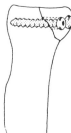
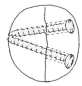

Fig. 2.131   Displaced fractures of the head of the radius and their reduction and fixation.

Fig. 2.132   Lateral and antero-posterior X-rays of a fracture of the radial head, showing perfect reduction and fixation using a Herbert screw.

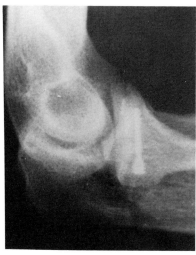
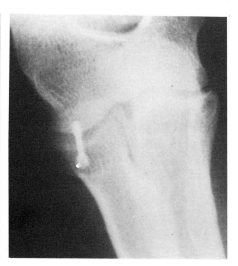

Comminuted fractures can often be reconstituted with care (Fig. 2.133). Those that can't be reconstituted, for example Fig. 2.134, require excision of the radial head.

Fig. 2.134   Antero-posterior X-ray of a grossly comminuted fracture of the head of the radius – this one will need excision.

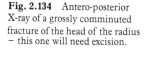
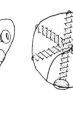
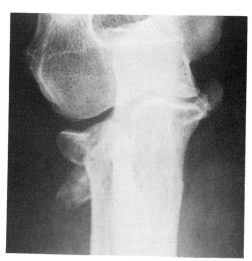

Fig. 2.133   Reconstruction of the radial head with multiple screws.

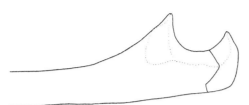 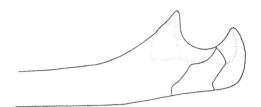

Fig. 2.135   Undisplaced fractures of the olecranon.

Olecranon

In both adults and children this fracture can be an isolated lesion or it can be associated with dislocation of the radial head as in a Monteggia fracture (see the section on **Monteggia's fracture ·dislocation of the forearm above**).

In undisplaced fractures (Fig. 2.135), the treatment will consist of immobilization in a long arm backslab for three weeks and the active but careful use of the arm for a further three weeks. The elbow movement will return rapidly and normal function can be expected.

This fracture will displace if it (the fracture) is complete, due to the strong action of the triceps muscle which is inserted into the olecranon. If it is displaced (Fig. 2.136) it will not reduce even if the arm is put in full extension. Therefore, open reduction and internal fixation will be necessary (Fig. 2.136). The fracture is often compound (or open) as the olecranon is subcutaneous.

Fig. 2.136   Displaced fractures of the olecranon and some techniques of internal fixation.

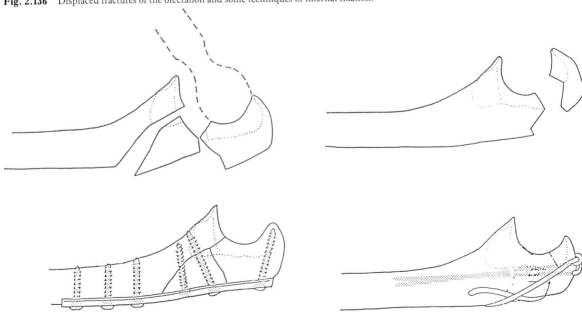

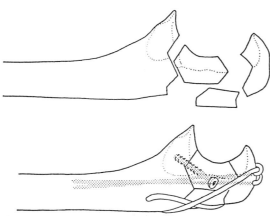

Fig. 2.137   This is an intra-articular fracture and the joint will need reconstruction.

Remember that this is *always* an intra-articular fracture and as such must be accurately reduced and firmly fixed (Fig. 2.137).

Distal end of the humerus

These are the T and Y shaped fractures (Fig. 2.138). This used to be called the 'baby car' fracture. In the days before mechanical signals, when the hands were used to indicate stop and turn, there was a gruesome saying:

> 'Don't put your hand out too far,
>   it may go home in another car.'

These were horrible compound injuries that are now less frequently seen. Compound injuries need special care (see the section on *Compound fractures* in Ch. 1 above).

Non-compound fractures of this type occur as a result of a fall on the point of the elbow. The ulna is driven, like a wedge, into the lower end of the humerus.

Fig. 2.138   Some of the T and Y shaped fractures of the distal humerus.

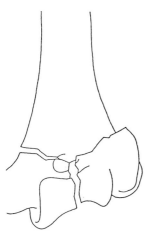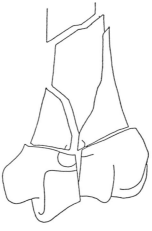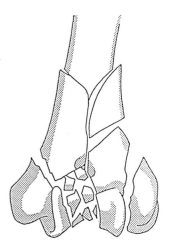

Treatment

1. Undisplaced fractures require six weeks in a padded backslab with the elbow at ninety degrees.

2. Closed reduction of the fracture by moulding and the application of a posterior slab is the classical treatment. However, the results are usually very poor since very little elbow movement is regained as a rule.

3. Active treatment, by ignoring the fracture and encouraging movement, gives better end results and even the X-rays often look surprisingly good. Put the arm in a collar and cuff initially and give the patient some strong analgesics.

4. The treatment of choice, **if the surgeon can carry out this difficult operation,** is to carry out open reduction and accurately fix the fragments with plates and screws. Initial treatment, whilst awaiting the operation, is a well padded backslab.

Shaft of the humerus – children and adults

Fractures of the shaft of the humerus (like all long bones) can be one of a number of types of fracture, namely:

Transverse – greenstick
Oblique
Spiral
Comminuted

Any of these, except perhaps the greenstick fracture, can be compound (see *Compound fractures* section in Ch. 1 above).

Transverse – greenstick

These are rare and are due to direct trauma in a young child. The cortex may be only buckled or broken on one side with some angulation (Fig. 2.139).

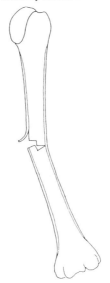

Fig. 2.139 Transverse fracture of the humerus caused by direct trauma.

Management

If there is significant angulation, it needs to be corrected by manipulation (usually under a general anaesthetic). Immobilization in the very young is by binding the arm to the thorax, but in an older child or an adult it is by a U-slab and bandage (Fig. 2.140).

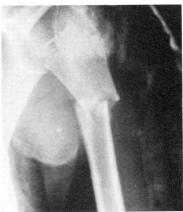

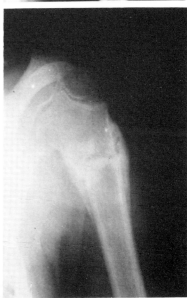

Fig. 2.140 Antero-posterior X-ray of a transverse fracture of the humerus in a U-slab and at four weeks.

HOW TO APPLY A U-SLAB

1. Measure the length of the slab to be used. It should run from the axilla down the inner surface of the arm, under the elbow, up the outer side of the arm and over the deltoid to the outer third of the clavicle.

2. Insert this slab (10 thicknesses of 15cm width plaster) into a wide piece of stockingette, twice as long as the slab.

3. Apply the slab over the padding by: wetting the stockingette and slab at the slab end only; then start at the axilla and go around the elbow and up over the shoulder — hold the arm with a crepe bandage; now tie the long end of the stockingette to the wrist after padding it with cotton wool or Velband where it passes around the neck.

The slab is self supporting (Fig. 2.141).

Fig. 2.141 This type of U-slab is self supporting.

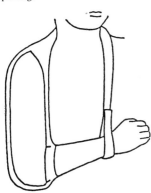

Transverse displaced

This fracture (Fig. 2.142) is usually due to direct trauma in a motor vehicle accident, or on the sporting field.

Management

Reduce the fracture under a general anaesthetic and if the fracture is stable, apply the U-slab as above.

Fig. 2.142 Displaced transverse fracture of the humerus.

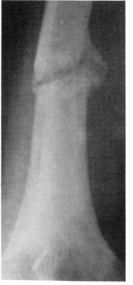

The patient will need to be X-rayed about every ten days to make sure that the position remains satisfactory — remember that whilst some displacement can be accepted (Fig. 2.143) because length is not critical, uncorrected angulation will lead to an ugly deformity. Remanipulate the fracture if necessary.

Fig. 2.143 Lateral and antero-posterior X-rays of a displaced transverse fracture of the humerus before reduction and some weeks later when uniting.

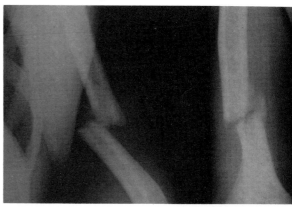

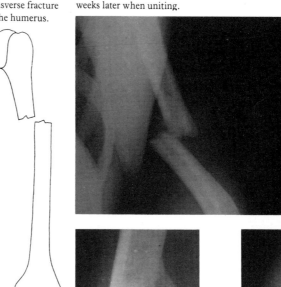

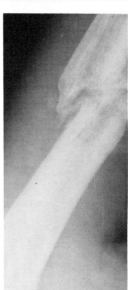

Oblique

These fractures are caused by direct violence. The fracture line usually runs distally and medially (Figs. 2.144a and b).

Fig. 2.144   Oblique fracture of the humerus.

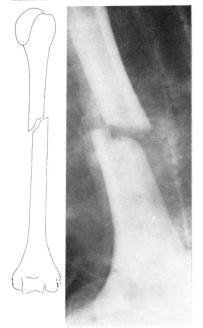

In oblique and spiral fractures always check the radial nerve to see if it has been damaged or even cut by a bone fragment. (The radial nerve runs in the spiral groove around the humerus and is therefore often damaged in oblique and spiral fractures.)

To test the function of the radial nerve ask the patient to extend the wrist (Fig. 2.145).

Fig. 2.145   Testing the radial nerve by active dorsiflexion of the wrist.

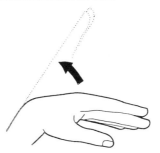

Management

Reduction of the fracture may require a general anaesthetic, but with traction on the arm and the patient sitting, moulding and direct pressure will usually reduce the fracture. Then apply a U-slab and X-ray in ten days. The slabs should be tightened at the same time.

It takes eight to ten weeks for this fracture to unite in an adult and about six weeks in a child.

Spiral fractures

Spiral fractures of the humerus (Fig. 2.146) are often the result of a fall on the extended arm or a twisting injury. These fractures *have muscle interposed if there is significant displacement (Fig. 2.147).*

Test the function of the radial nerve – Ask the patient to extend their wrist (Fig. 2.145).

Fig. 2.146
Spiral fracture of the humerus.

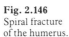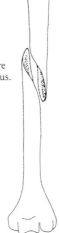

Fig. 2.147   Spiral fracture of the humerus with muscle interposition.

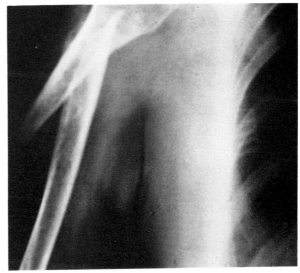

Management

Closed reduction should be tried
where possible. Again have the
patient seated with the arm
hanging, then with traction mould
the fracture (Fig. 2.148) and apply a
U-slab. Open reduction is necessary
when muscle is interposed (Fig.
2.147).

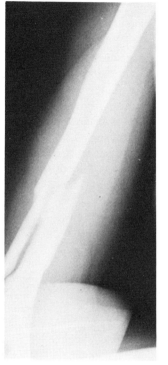
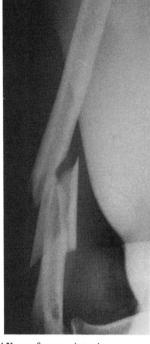

Fig. 2.148 Antero-posterior X-ray of a well
reduced spiral fracture of the humerus.

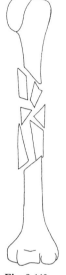

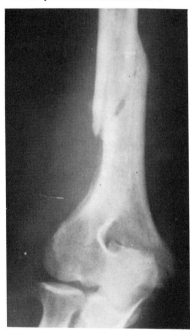

Fig. 2.149
Comminuted
fracture of the
humerus.

Fig. 2.150 Antero-posterior and lateral X-ray of a comminuted
fracture of the humerus.

Fig. 2.151 Post operative X-rays showing
union of the comminuted fracture of the
humerus shown in Figure 2.150.

Comminuted

These are rare. They result from
direct violence and may be
compound (Figs. 2.149 and 2.150).

Management

Closed fractures can often be
manipulated into good positions and
be treated by immobilization in a U-
slab. **If a good position is not
obtained, open reduction
should be carried out (Fig.
2.151).**

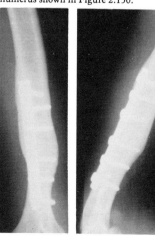

Fractures of the humerus with radial nerve paralysis. Clinically, radial nerve palsy is easily detected:

1. **The patient has wrist drop (Fig. 2.152).**

Fig. 2.152 Wrist drop with no active dorsiflexion.

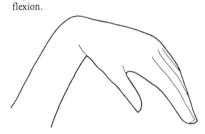

2. **There is sensory loss on the dorsum of the hand near the thumb (Fig. 2.153).**

Fig. 2.153 The area of anaesthesia in a radial nerve lesion.

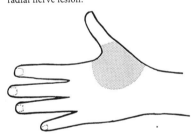

The radial nerve is usually bruised rather than cut and over 90 per cent

Fig. 2.154 A cock-up splint.

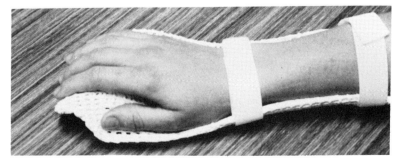

of the lesions recover within two months.

The nerve can be cut by a sharp fragment or by a penetrating object in open fractures.

Treatment

1. Treat the fractured humerus according to the methods discussed on previous page.

2. In open fractures, the nerve should be visualised, and if it is intact, nothing further needs to be done – the nerve will recover. If the nerve is severed, **microsurgical repair is necessary.**

3. In closed fractures, the nerve can be assumed to be suffering from neuropraxia and this can usually be confirmed by e.m.g. testing. If this is so, then all that needs to be done is to support the wrist at night in a 'cock-up' splint (Fig. 2.154) and ask the patient to exercise passively the wrist and fingers hourly during the day.

4. Occasionally the nerve gets caught in the callus and fails to recover. In this case or if the nerve has not shown signs of recovery on e.m.g. or clinically in 8-10 weeks, exploration is indicated.

Sensory recovery precedes motor recovery by two to three weeks.

Neck and head of the humerus

This is a fracture that is common in the elderly, and is usually not displaced significantly (Figs. 2.155 and 2.156).

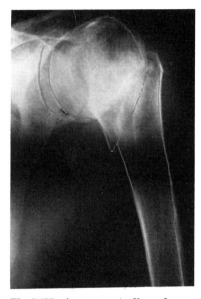

Fig. 2.155 Antero-posterior X-ray of a fracture of the neck of the humerus.

Fig. 2.156 Antero-posterior X-ray of a comminuted but indisplaced fracture of the neck of the humerus in an elderly lady.

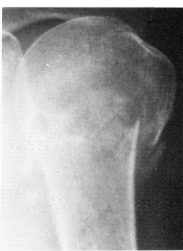

Undisplaced fractures require immobilization in an inside collar and cuff with an axillary pad. Advise the patient and relatives to keep the arm inside the clothes for one week. During this time extensive bruising will appear – warn the patient of this or they will be frightened at its appearance. After one week, very gentle exercise can begin and the arm can be kept outside the clothes. Physiotherapy is often required at the two to three week stage.

Displaced fractures of the neck of the humerus may require open reduction and internal fixation (Fig. 2.157), especially in the younger of the elderly group that suffer this fracture.

Comminuted and displaced fractures of the neck and head of the humerus may require reconstruction (Fig. 2.158) or even replacement.

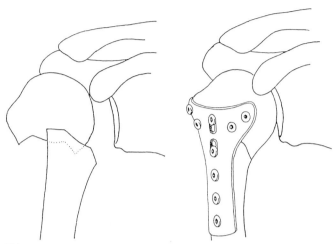

Fig. 2.157(a)   Displaced fracture of the neck of the humerus in a young person; and **(b)** its open reduction.

Fig. 2.158   Comminuted fracture of the head of the humerus with displacement.

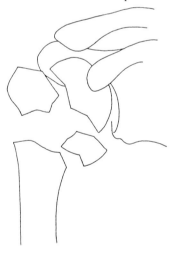

CHAPTER THREE

Fractures and dislocations of the trunk

Fractures of the clavicle

Probably the commonest injury during childhood is the fracture of the clavicle in its middle third (Fig. 3.1). The fracture is usually caused by a fall onto an outstretched hand. Football injuries are another common cause.

Greenstick

By definition these are incomplete fractures with bending at the fracture site (Fig. 3.2). Most birth fractures and those up to the age of six are of this type, as the periosteum is tougher than in older children and adults.

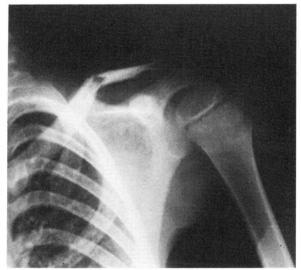

Fig. 3.1   Incomplete fracture of the clavicle in its middle third.

Fig 3.2   Incomplete fracture of the clavicle at ten days.

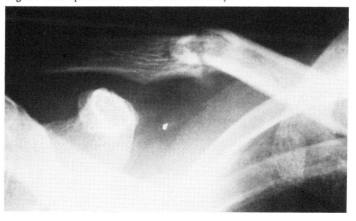

Management

Immobilization of the arm in a sling under the clothes is all that is necessary. Warn the parents that in the young child a large lump of callus will appear at the fracture site in a few weeks and remould over the next few months. Parents tend not to believe you if you try to tell them this after the lump has appeared, but realise that you know what you are talking about if you forewarn them.

Use the sling under the clothes for the first two weeks and then outside the clothes. Discard the sling when the fracture is no longer tender to pressure but avoid sport for a further three weeks.

Displaced

Whilst some authorities on the subject suggest that you accept the deformity (Fig. 3.3) and the resultant malunion with its prominent bony lump, others do not – hence treatment of this injury depends on which school of thought your hospital and orthopaedic consultants follow.

Fig. 3.3   Displaced fracture of the middle third of the clavicle – no bump.

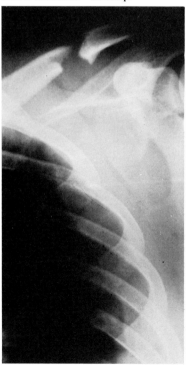

1. *The pessimists.* These people maintain that some degree of malunion is inevitable, and that you should accept the bump (Fig. 3.4). They advise you to simply put the patient in a sling for a few weeks and encourage active use of the arm after three weeks.

2. *The optimists.* They maintain that the fracture can be reduced by the application of a 'figure of eight' or 'rucksack' type of splint (Fig. 3.5).

Those opposed to this type of treatment point out, that if the system is pulled too tight the

Fig. 3.4   Displaced fracture of the clavicle with a bump.

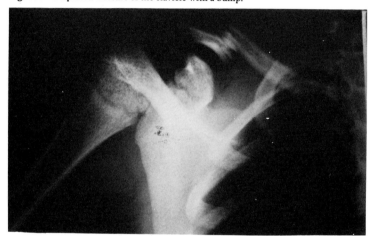

circulation in the arms can be compromised by pressure on the axillary vessels − moving the arms out from the sides will relieve this.

The system needs to be tightened frequently, every second day, for three weeks − this can be done by the parents − and then the arm used carefully for a further three weeks.

So the choice of treatment is yours!

How to apply the figure of eight type splint

Measure and fit a tight loop of stockingette filled with foam around the back of the neck and under the arms as shown in the first two diagrams. Then arch the shoulders back and tie the loops together (Fig. 3.6).

I believe that film stars have their fractures of the clavicle treated by lying flat on their backs in bed with a sandbag between the shoulder blades. In this position the fracture comes together and there should be no bump on the clavicle to spoil their beauty.

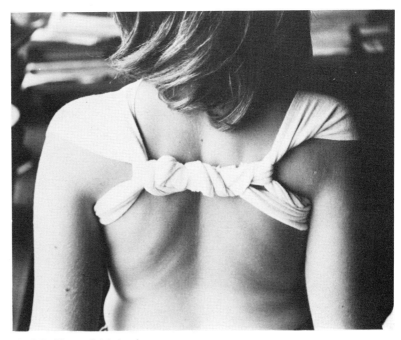

Fig. 3.5 Figure of eight bandage.

Fig. 3.6 Steps in applying a figure of eight bandage.

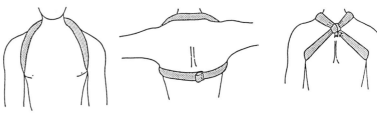

Fractures of the scapula

Scapular fractures are rare and usually the result of direct trauma. The scapula is well covered with muscles and tends to crack rather than to shatter (Fig. 3.7).

Fig. 3.7   Crack fractures of the scapula.

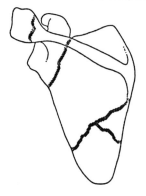

Any part of the scapula can be fractured. Provided that it is an undisplaced crack fracture (Figs. 3.8 and 3.9) and the glenoid is not involved, there are no problems.

Management

A sling is all that is necessary. However, the arm will remain painful for about six weeks.

Displaced fractures of the acromion will need open reduction and fixation with K-wires or screws.

Fractures of the glenoid margin are very rare and may require operative treatment because the shoulder may become unstable (Figs. 3.10 and 3.11).

Fig. 3.8   Slightly displaced fracture of the scapula.

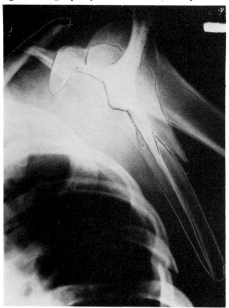

Fig. 3.9   Undisplaced but complete fracture of the body of the scapula.

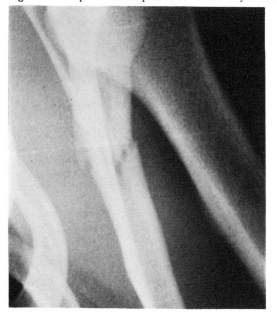

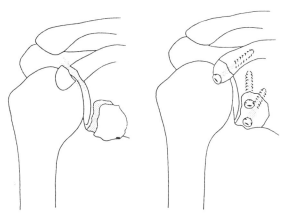

Fig. 3.10   Unstable fracture of the glenoid margin — screw fixation.

Fig. 3.11   Unstable fracture of the glenoid margin — plate fixation.

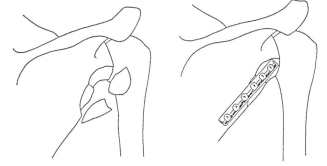

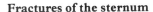

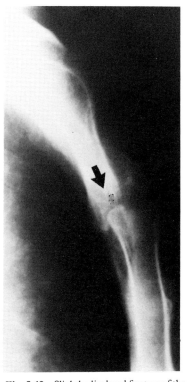

Fig. 3.12   Slightly displaced fracture of the sternum.

Fractures of the sternum

Motor vehicle accidents are the main cause of this problem. Prior to the advent and use of seat belts, the sternum was fractured on the steering wheel. Now in high speed injuries, the seat belt itself can be the cause of damage to the sternum, ribs and the liver — without the seat belt these people would be killed.

The most common type of injury is a fracture at or near the manubrium (Fig. 3.12).

You must be careful in examining this patient. This can be an isolated injury — but it may be part of a more serious chest, abdominal and thoracic spine injury.

All patients require admission and monitoring (respiration and E.C.G.) for twenty-four hours.

Displaced fractures probably have an underlying myocardial contusion — beware of cardiac tamponade.

The sternal injury itself requires no special treatment, but it is painful and the patient will need analgesics and care to avoid direct pressure over the injury.

Indications for treatment of the bony injury are pain and deformity. Operative treatment is extremely rare.

Fractures of the ribs

Most rib fractures are caused by direct injuries, such as hitting the chest on the corner of a piece of furniture. Fractures can occur as a result of stress − by muscular action or even by severe coughing. Seat belt injuries are also common.

The ribs are well covered by muscles and seldom displace. They tend to fracture at the angle (Fig. 3.13). **When there is displacement, the rib often punctures the pleura or lung causing a haemothorax, a pneumothorax, or both.**

Fig. 3.13   Displaced fractures of the ribs.

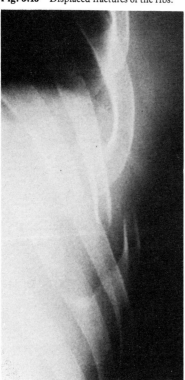

The patient who has had a chest injury and who is unable to expand the chest in spite of a clear airway has a pneumothorax or haemopneumothorax until proven otherwise. **A tension pneumothorax has positive pressure in the pleural cavity and will require urgent release of the pressure by drainage to relieve a rapidly worsening respiratory status.**

For simple rib fractures, the clinical picture is clear − local tenderness over the fracture site with stabbing pain on deep breathing and pain on compression of the thorax.

X-rays will confirm the diagnosis.

Management

Analgesics are important, as are instructions on deep breathing. Strapping the chest is seldom advised nowadays, as it is felt that this discourages deep breathing. The ribs unite spontaneously and are painful during breathing for three weeks and to touch for several months.

The use of long acting local anaesthetic (such as one per cent Marcaine) has its advocates in those patients who have so much pain that they simply will *not* breathe deeply. This is not a technique for general use in casualty. If it is used, care needs to be taken: to maintain sterility; to avoid creating a pneumothorax; and to avoid injecting the Marcaine into a vessel.

Beware of the patient with multiple fractured ribs as they often have underlying pulmonary damage and, because of pain, need to have supervised breathing exercises to prevent atelectasis and infection.

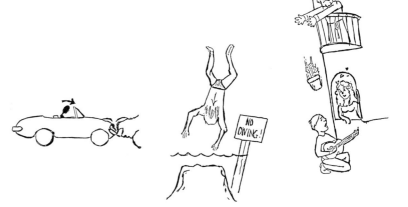

Fig. 3.14   The common causes of injury to the cervical spine.

Fractures and fracture dislocations of the spine

Cervical vertebrae

A subject of great presage: if you miss such a fracture dislocation then the patient could become **paraplegic**; and if you badly manage a partial paralysis, it may become **complete!**

The key factors in proper treatment are:

1. **Suspect the injury**
2. **Recognize the problem on X-ray**
3. **Adequate initial care.**

1. Suspect the injury

You must suspect that a cervical spine injury has occurred in the unconscious patient who has been in an accident. The head after all, is attached to the neck and any violence to the head could also cause neck damage. It is therefore important that all unconscious patients with head injuries have X-rays of the cervical spine.

All conscious patients who have neck pain will need X-rays, after clinical assessment and perhaps the use of a collar (see Ch. 8, Fig. 8.27). Look very carefully at injuries due to: motor vehicle accidents; those who fall from a height onto their heads; those who are hit on the head or neck; and those who dive into shallow water.

Do not hesitate to have X-rays done again if the patient is in severe pain, or has neurological signs of spinal cord damage.

Tomography and computerised axial tomography will sometimes be of great help, particularly in the atlanto-axial region.

2. Recognize the problem on X-ray

X-rays of the cervical spine in an injured patient often do not show the entire area you need to see.

You must check down to C7 in the lateral view, otherwise you can miss a C6-7 dislocation – a not infrequent injury.

Fig. 3.15 Cervical spine X-rays, antero-posterior, lateral and oblique.

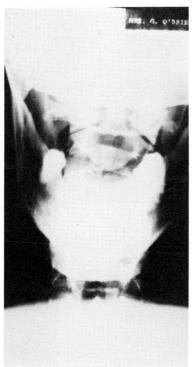 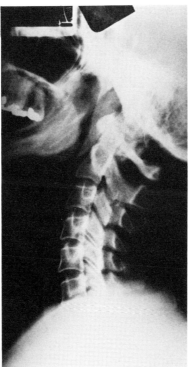 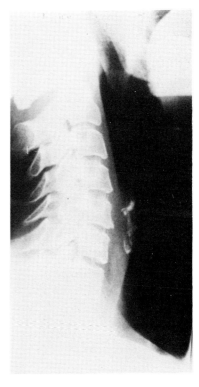

Look at the X-rays in Fig. 3.15 – are they normal?

Yes, they are. Now look at the films systematically to be sure we have not overlooked any injury.

Make sure that you can see C7 and also the odontoid process.

Look at the films in Figure 3.16.

Note that I have drawn in lines along the anterior and posterior margins of the vertebral bodies in the lateral view and that these lines are not broken and that the cervical spine has its normal curve (lordosis).

Now check the outline of each vertebral body to see there are no chipped margins or crushed edges.

Now check the odontoid process both on the lateral and antero-posterior view – look at the arrow.

Finally check the spinous processes and the transverse processes.

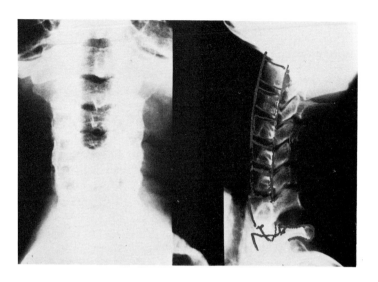

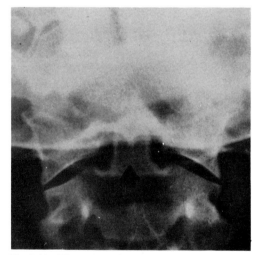

Fig. 3.16   The method of checking the antero-posterior, lateral and oblique X-rays of the cervical spine.

Try again with Figures 3.17, 3.18a and b.

Figures 3.19 to 3.22 are further examples of the many types of injury to the cervical spine. All of them are serious or potentially serious.

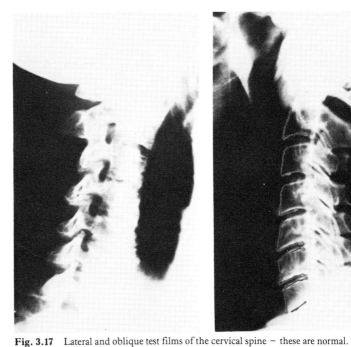
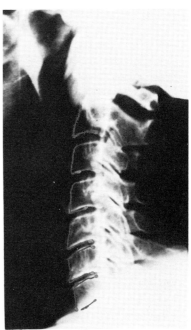

Fig. 3.17   Lateral and oblique test films of the cervical spine − these are normal.

Fig. 3.18(a)   Diagram of a C5–6 dislocation; **(b)** Lateral X-ray showing a C4–5 dislocation.

Fig. 3.19   Fracture of the lamina and spinous process of C2 with displacement.

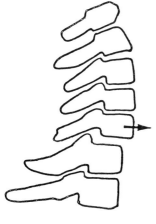
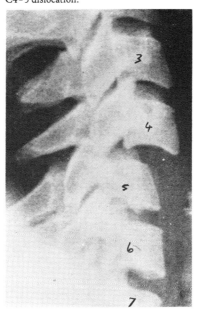
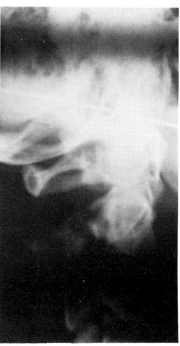

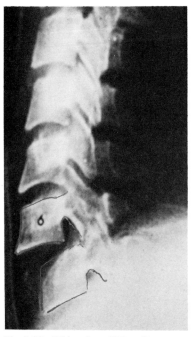

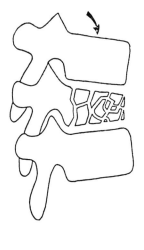

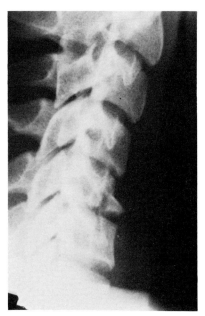

Fig. 3.22   Crush fracture of C5.

Fig. 3.20   Dislocation of C6 on C7.

Fig. 3.21   Fracture of the odontoid process of C2.

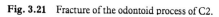

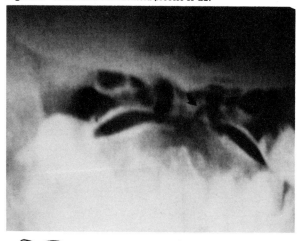

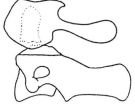

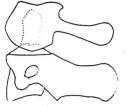

Initial care

1. At the accident site, make sure that all suspected neck injuries are looked after carefully and the neck is not flexed or extended – if possible apply a collar.

2. As soon as possible after the patient arrives in casualty, he or she will need to be assessed clinically. If they are complaining of neck pain, exercise extreme care in moving either the neck or the patient until X-rays have been done.

Examine the patient neurologically to see if there is any loss of motor power, sensation or reflexes in the limbs.

Any loss of power, sensation or reflexes, indicates a serious injury – **apply a collar (Fig. 3.23) before sending to the X-ray department. Go with the patient, and supervise movement during the X-rays.**

If the X-rays are normal and pain is severe, arrange admission for further treatment.

If the X-rays appear normal but there is paralysis, sensory and reflex loss, this indicates spinal cord damage and it will be necessary to transfer the patient to the spinal unit. The patient must be immobilized in a collar, handled very gently and accompanied by a doctor.

If the X-rays are not normal, you must assess them correctly (as we have already discussed) and decide if the lesion is a stable one.

Stable fractures (Fig. 3.24) need admission for observation, analgesics and rest in a support.

Unstable lesions and dislocations (Fig. 3.25) will need expert help because you will need to apply skull traction and reduce any dislocation.

Fig. 3.23   The initial care of a suspected cervical spine injury.

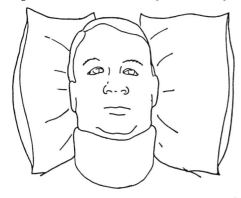

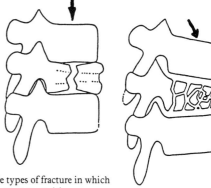

Fig. 3.24   Stable types of fracture in which the spinal cord is not at great risk.

Fig. 3.25   Unstable fractures, in which the spinal cord may be damaged and is at risk.

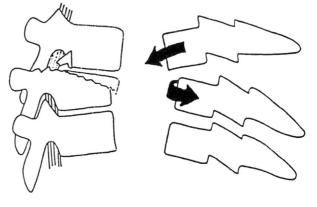

Thoracic vertebrae

These fractures are common in elderly patients, where they are associated with demineralisation of the vertebrae and often occur with minimal trauma.

In younger people, severe trauma is needed to cause fractures and fracture dislocations are almost always associated with paraplegia.

1. *Suspect the injury*

In high speed motor vehicle accidents; workers involved in cave-in accidents, such as miners (Fig. 3.26); and elderly people with much more minor trauma.

2. *Recognize the problem on X-ray*

Look at the X-ray of the thoracic spine (Fig. 3.27).

Is it normal?

No, it is not. Let's look at the X-rays using the same system as in the cervical spine.

Draw lines along the anterior and posterior vertebral margins (at least with your eye). Is there any break in these lines indicating a dislocation?

Next look around the margins of each vertebral body — they should be rectangular. Is there a crush fracture? Yes, there is a crush fracture of T10.

Here are some other X-rays of the thoracic spine, for you to look at systematically and to work out the diagnosis — see Figures 3.28 to 3.30 inclusive.

Fig. 3.26 Common causes of thoracic spine injuries.

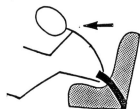
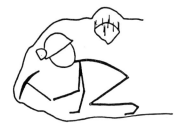

Fig. 3.27 Lateral view of the thoracic spine — a crush fracture is present.

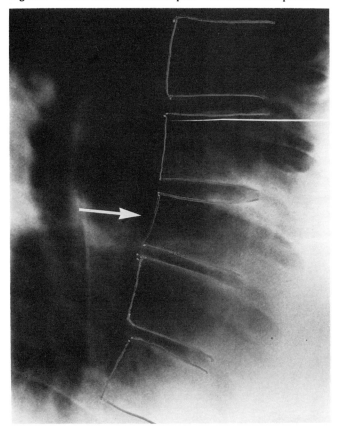

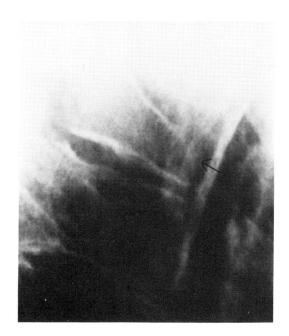

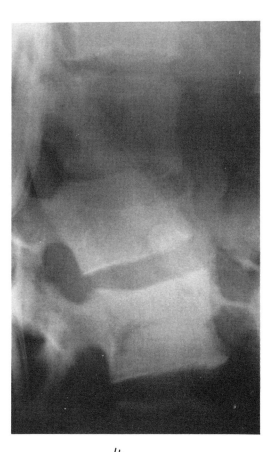

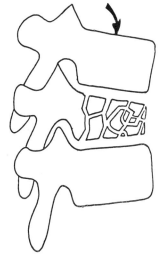

Fig. 3.28 X-ray and diagram of an extensive, stable, crush fracture of T4. A steel lid weighing one tonne fell on his neck and back.

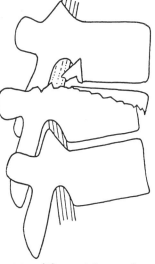

Fig. 3.29 A lateral X-ray and diagram of an unstable, slicing, fracture of a lower thoracic vertebrae.

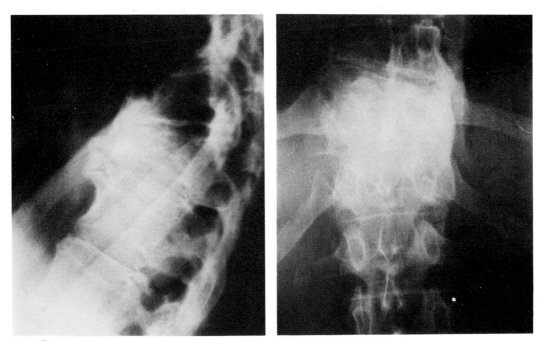

Fig. 3.30   Lateral and antero-posterior X-rays of pathological crush fractures.

Not all abnormally shaped vertebrae are the result of trauma, for example, see Fig. 3.31b. **This is not multiple crush fractures.** It is a developmental condition called **Scheuermann's disease**. This is an X-ray of a young patient and there will usually be no history of trauma (unless a patient with Scheuermann's disease is injured).

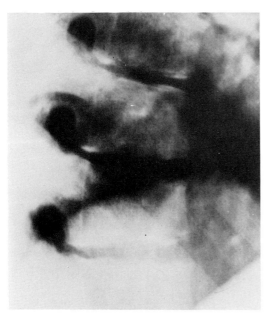

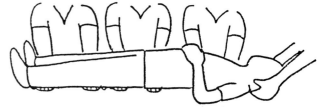

Fig. 3.31 (a)   How to move a patient with spinal injuries. Always support the spine so that it is neither flexed or extended.
(b)   Lateral X-ray of thoracic spine with Scheuermann's Disease.

3. *Initial care*

The patient will need to be moved with care, both from the scene of the accident and within the hospital – this means supporting the patient's spine on a rigid surface, so that the spine is neither flexed nor extended (Fig. 3.31a).

Examine the patient carefully, checking not only the neurological status but also looking for abdominal and chest injuries.

If there are neurological abnormalities, handle the patient with great care and go with the patient to the X-ray department.

Assess the X-rays as above and decide if the lesion is of the stable or unstable variety.

If the patient has a stable lesion with neurological problems, transfer to a special unit. It is, of course, much less likely that there will be problems if the lesion is a stable one. The presence of any serious neurological deficit means the cord has been damaged. Are you sure this is a stable lesion?

Stable lesions (Fig. 3.32), without neurological problems will need admission and bed rest for a week or so, followed by a rehabilitation programme. Some orthopaedic surgeons use a Taylor brace for a few weeks.

Fig. 3.32 Stable crush fractures.

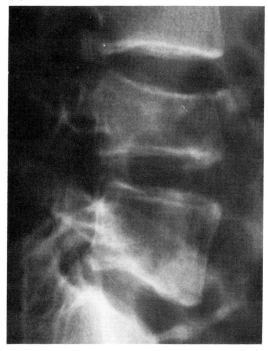
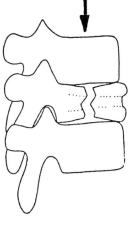
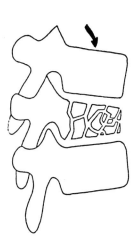

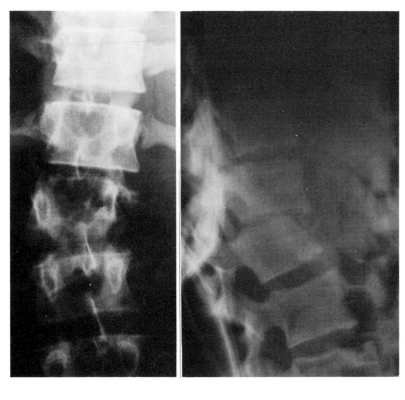

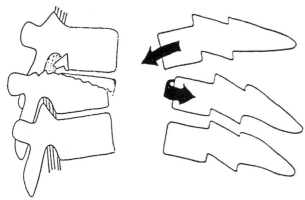

Fig. 3.33   Unstable fractures of the thoracic spine.

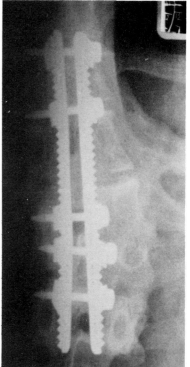

Unstable lessions (Fig. 3.33a and b) with partial paraplegia need to be transported to a special unit with extreme care.

Unstable lesions, without neurological problems, will need to be handled carefully until the lesion is stabilised surgically (Fig. 3.34).

Fig. 3.34   Surgical stabilisation of an unstable lower thoracic spine injury.

Lumbar vertebrae

These fractures are reasonably common. However, there is less frequent involvement of the spinal cord with neurological problems, than with injuries in the cervical and thoracic area.

1. *Suspect the injury*

Fractures of the lumbar spine occur most often as a result of a fall from a height. The other common injury in this type of fall is a fracture of the os calcis.

Motor vehicle accidents, particularly high speed ones, where a lap type seat belt is worn can cause a slicing type fracture of L1 (Chance fracture).

Direct injury to the spine, by a fall onto an object or the falling of an object onto the lumbar spine, can cause fractures of the transverse processes.

2. *Recognize the fracture*

The same principles should be applied here, as in the thoracic and cervical region. Please refer to the relevant sections on the preceding pages. Then examine the X-rays in the pattern suggested − alignment, shape of vertebrae, spinous and transverse processes.

3. *Initial care*

Again this depends on the presence or absence of neurological damage and whether the lesion is stable. Please refer back to the section on injuries to the thoracic vertebrae.

In summary:

a. If it is stable (Fig. 3.35) with paralysis − send the patient to a special unit.

b. If stable with no paralysis − send the patient to a ward for rest and analgesics.

Fig. 3.35 Stable crush fracture of the lumbar spine.

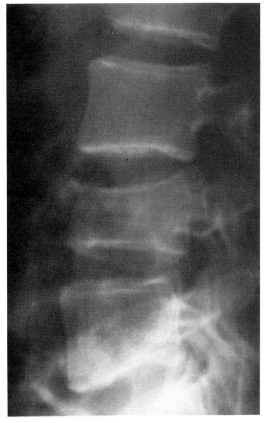
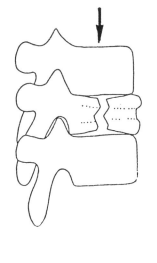
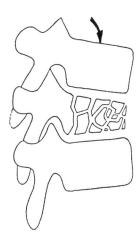

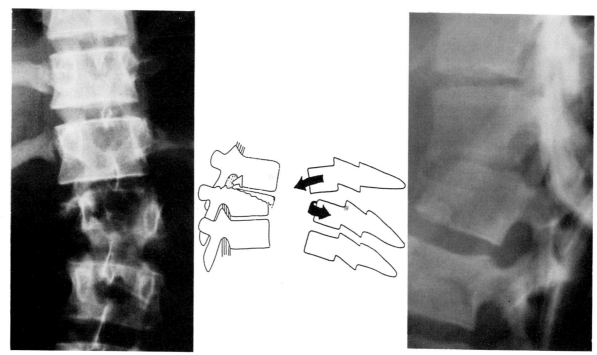

Fig. 3.36   Unstable fracture dislocation of T12-L1.

c. If unstable (Fig. 3.36a, b and c) with paralysis — send to a special unit with care.

d. If unstable without paralysis — send to a ward, with great care, until stabilized.

Fractures of the lumbar transverse processes (Fig. 3.37) can occur as a direct injury and, as such, there may also be damage to the kidneys — check the urine for blood. There may be considerable retroperitoneal bleeding, causing blood loss and shock and frequently a temporary paralytic ileus.

These fractures are not serious, but they are painful. The patients usually need admission to hospital for bed rest and analgesics for a few days, followed by physiotherapy treatment in the form of heat and exercises.

Fig. 3.37   Multiple fractures of the transverse processes of the lumbar vertebrae.

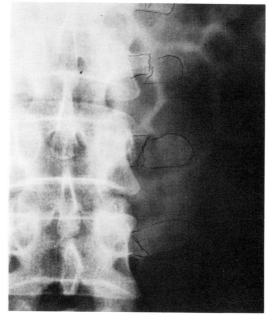

Sacrum and coccyx

A fall on the ice is not common in Australia but it is common in other countries and often causes a crack fracture of the sacrum (Fig. 3.38) or of the coccyx (Fig. 3.39). displacement of the fractured sacrum and damage to the cauda equina is rare.

In fact, in this country, a fall down steps is the commonest cause of this injury, but it can also be caused by any other fall or direct blow to the area (such as a hard kick).

These fractures are painful, particularly whilst sitting and travelling in public transport.

Apart from the pain and the indignity of having to eat off the mantel shelf or carry around an 'air ring', this injury usually presents no special problems.

An air ring is like a child's flotation ring for the swimming pool, only your patient sits the tender bottom in the centre of the ring, and the air filled ring keeps the tender part away from pressure.

Pain and discomfort on sitting are usually severe for about three weeks and gradually fades over about three months.

Occasionally persistent pain or deformity in the coccygeal region necessitates operative removal of the coccyx.

Fig. 3.38 Slightly displaced fracture of the sacrum.

Fig. 3.39 Fracture of the coccyx.

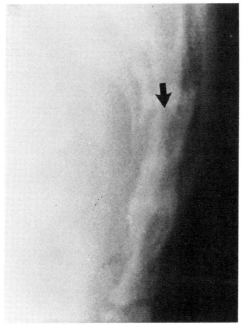

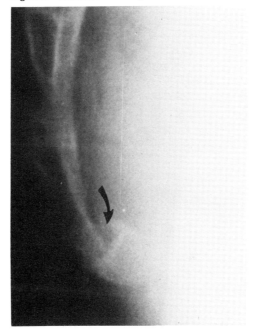

Fractures of the pelvis

The pelvis together with the sacrum forms a circle and whilst isolated pieces can be pulled off the ring of the pelvis, a displaced fracture at one point must have a corresponding fracture at another point (Fig. 3.40) or a dislocation – for example, of the sacro-iliac joint (Fig. 3.41).

The injury commonly occurs as a result of a motor vehicle accident; but falls from a height, crush injuries and even very simple falls in the elderly, can cause pelvic fractures. Some avulsion type fractures in young people are caused by muscular action.

About half of the patients who have major pelvic fractures have multiple injuries to other structures, some of which will prove fatal – such as head injuries. Many have significant injuries to the pelvic organs and to the soft tissues around the pelvis.

The associated complications – namely extensive haemorrhage and shock, and extravasation of urine from bladder or urethral injuries – are often more important than the fracture of the pelvis itself.

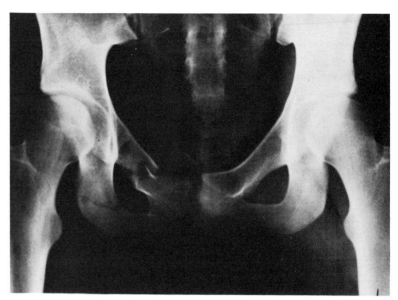

Fig. 3.40   Double fracture of the pubis.

Fig. 3.41   Fractures of the pubis and dislocation of the sacro-iliac joint on the same side.

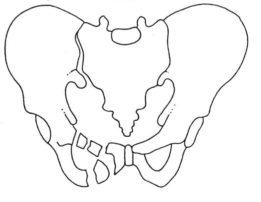

Initial care

The patient needs to be assessed carefully to ascertain the extent of the injuries. Is this just local bony damage? Beware of the patient with a pelvic fracture who becomes shocked quickly – they are usually bleeding freely in the pelvis or abdomen.

In any seriously injured or shocked patient, your first priority is to set up an intravenous drip and to send off blood for cross-matching. **Displacement of the pubic bones, by disruption (Fig. 3.42) or fracture (Fig. 3.43), is often associated with visceral injury.** The common internal organ that is damaged in pelvic fractures is the bladder, so this needs to be checked.

Checklist:

1. Find out, if possible, when the patient last passed urine – an empty bladder is less likely to have been damaged.

2. If the patient can void and there is plenty of clear urine, then there is no evidence of bladder injury.

3. If the patient is unable to void (and this is often due to pain), then catheterise the patient. Failure to pass a catheter usually indicates a ruptured urethra – a urethrogram will confirm.

4. If the catheter is easily passed and the urine is clear, then there is no injury.

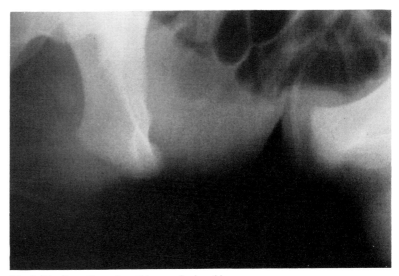

Fig. 3.42   Gross disruption of the symphysis pubis.

Fig. 3.43   Fracture of the ischium involving the hip joint – the bladder is intact and full of dye.

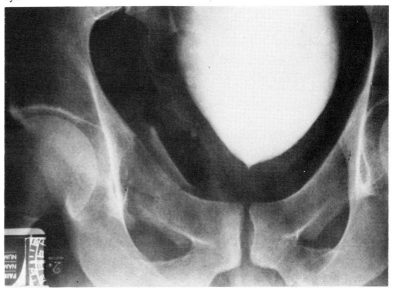

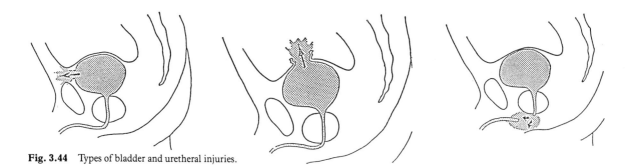

Fig. 3.44   Types of bladder and uretheral injuries.

5. A very small amount of heavily bloodstained urine may indicate an extra-peritoneal rupture of the bladder, usually by a spike of bone. A large volume of bloodstained urine indicates bladder damage – a cystogram with emptying will help you work out the problem.

Patients with bladder or urethral injuries (Fig. 3.44) will, of course, need admission to the hospital for definitive treatment of the urological problem – organize admission, then blood for transfusion (if necessary) and theatre time.

Treatment of the fracture takes second place to the treatment of the other more serious injuries. Internal fixation of the pelvic fractures can rarely be carried out during the same operation. The pelvic fractures are usually treated by bed rest or, if they are of the displaced type, by traction as described on the following pages.

Isolated and avulsed

There are many fractures of the pelvis that are not displaced (Fig. 3.45), or are minimally displaced (Fig. 3.46) and require minimal treatment.

Fig. 3.45   Undisplaced fracture of the floor of the acetabulum.

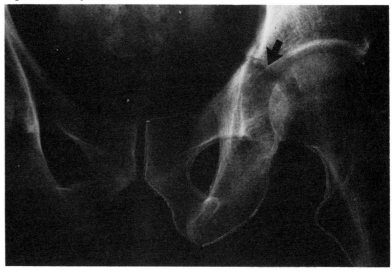

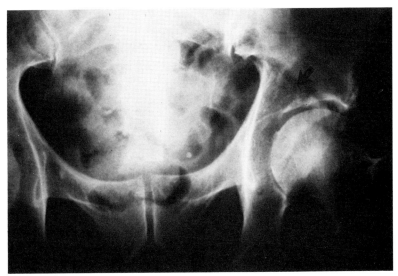

Fig. 3.46   Minimally displaced fracture of the iliac bone involving the hip joint.

These fractures are not associated with visceral injuries and require symptomatic treatment only.

Generally patients with undisplaced fractures and no other injuries can be managed by bed rest for a few days and then graduated activity for a few weeks.

Occasionally an avulsion fracture (Fig. 3.47) requires reattachment of the avulsed fragment, but usually these injuries are treated by rest and support of the limb.

With disruption of the acetabulum

See *Dislocations of the hip* in Chapter 5.

Fig. 3.47   Avulsion fracture of the ischial tuberosity.

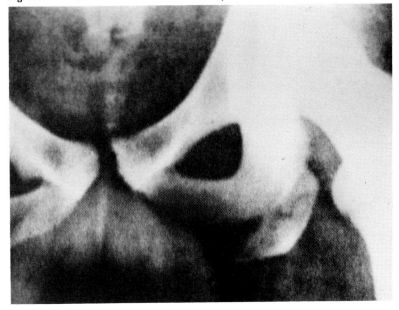

Fractures of the pelvis with disruption of the pelvic ring

Some examples of these are shown in Figures 3.48 and 3.49. As you can see, these types of disruptions allow one limb and half of the pelvis to ride up and the limb to shorten.

Disruption of the symphysis (Figs. 3.50 and 3.51) can vary from minor to the gross disruption of Figure 3.51.

Treatment of the bony injury will include reduction, if possible, and strong traction usually through skeletal traction from a tibial Steinman or Denham pin. Details of how to insert this pin and set up the traction are dealt with under treatment of *Fractures of the femur* in Chapter 6.

Internal fixation of fractures of the pelvis is advocated by some orthopaedic surgeons − it is bold and bloody surgery and is not for the faint hearted or *inexperienced* surgeon.

External fixation (Fig. 3.52) is of great value in disruptions of the pelvis, and is not difficult to insert.

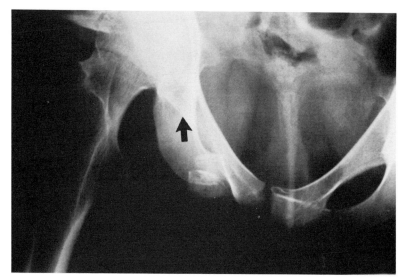

Fig. 3.48   Fracture of the pelvis with proximal shift of one side of the pelvis.

Fig. 3.49   Fracture of the pelvis with gross disruption of the sacro-iliac joint.

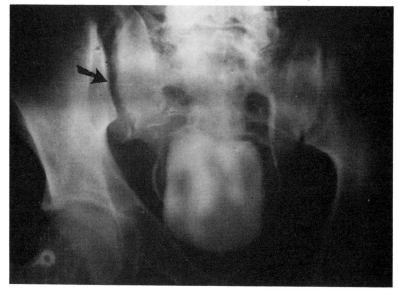

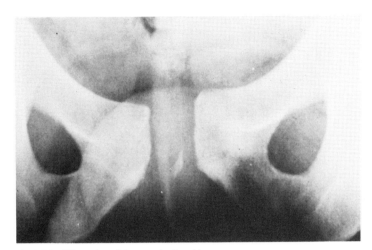

Fig. 3.50   Disruption of the symphysis pubis.

Fig. 3.51   Gross disruption of the symphysis pubis.

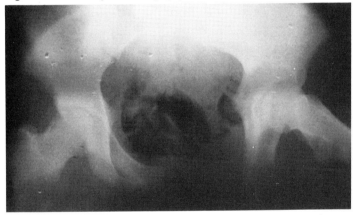

Fig. 3.52   External fixation in place on a bony pelvic skeleton, using the Hoffman apparatus.

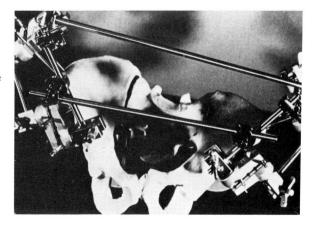

CHAPTER FOUR

Fractures of the lower limb

Fractures of the femur

The neck – adults

You will find that most N.O.F.'s are L.O.L.'s! Translated into English that means that most patients with fractures of the **n**eck **o**f the **f**emur are **l**ittle **o**ld **l**adies. (Just as most patients with fractures of the neck of the humerus are L.O.L.'s.)

The injury occurs when the patient stumbles and falls. This is often due to a minor cerebro-vascular episode, which probably accounts for the deterioration in their condition on admission to hospital, compared to that at home or in the nursing home.

The injury can occur in younger people with more violent injuries, but it is much more common in people in their late sixties, seventies and eighties. It is not uncommon to have a patient who is over ninety and who has previously suffered a fracture of the other hip some years earlier.

The clinical diagnosis is not difficult, as you have the following: an elderly person who has fallen; the complaint of pain in the groin; and the affected leg is shortened and

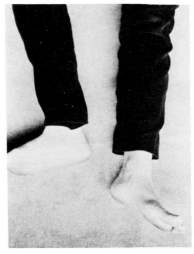

Fig. 4.1 Shortening and external rotation – signs of a fractured neck of the femur in an elderly person.

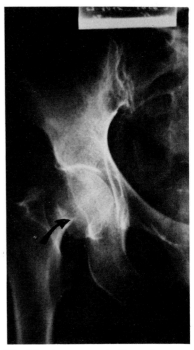

Fig. 4.2 Antero-posterior X-ray of a fractured neck of femur.

externally rotated (see Fig. 4.1) – except where the fracture is impacted.

On the X-rays (Fig. 4.2), the neck just does not run into the head – look particularly at the lower border of the neck and trace the line of the calcar femorale up to the head. This line ends and does not continue onto the lower border of the head when a fracture is present.

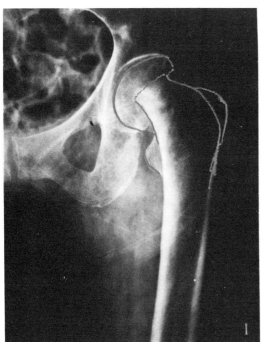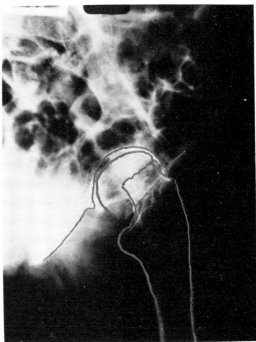

Fig. 4.3   Antero-posterior and lateral X-ray of an impacted fracture of the neck of the femur.

Naturally the patient will be admitted to hospital and, with the exception of the impacted fracture, will require an operation – if they are fit enough.

What the orthopaedic surgeon will need to know from the casualty officer will be:

1. Is the fracture impacted? (No operation if it is.)

2. How fit is this patient for an operation?

3. With what type of fracture are we dealing?

1. Is the fracture impacted?

Clinically, this is also easy to determine. Is the leg externally rotated and shortened (see Fig. 4.1)? If it is, then the fracture cannot be impacted and you are being deceived by overlap on the X-rays.

The fracture shown in Figure 4.3 is impacted and the leg of this patient would not be externally rotated. You would be able to put the hip through a fair range of movement without pain.

Some surgeons operate on all these fractures, as they say they dis-impact all too frequently, while others will leave them to have bed rest in hospital for two or three weeks.

2. How fit is this patient for operation?

We are dealing with a very fragile group. These elderly people, especially if they have been bedridden in a nursing home, will often have severe cardiac and pulmonary disease. They will need to be examined for cardiac, respiratory and renal function and, of course, will need a full blood analysis. Even so, if it is possible, these patients are better with the fracture actively dealt with than lying in bed where they will only succumb to pressure sores and respiratory infections.

3. *What type of fracture?*

Whilst an operation is necessary in almost all fractures of the neck of the femur, the actual procedure differs for different types of fracture. Figure 4.4 shows the neck as a stippled area and the trochanteric region as a striped area. The fractures that occur in the neck near the head are called subcapital fractures; lower down in the neck, they are called transcervical fractures; and in the striped area, they are called inter-trochanteric fractures.

The type of operation is dictated by the site of the fracture, and the age and activity level of the patient.

case is put on the next available routine operating list, it gives time for the tests to be done and the patient to be carefully examined by all concerned (including the anaesthetist and the social worker).

On admission to the ward and whilst awaiting operation, the patient needs to be put in either simple straight traction (Fig. 4.5), or Hamilton Russell traction (Figs. 4.15 and 4.16).

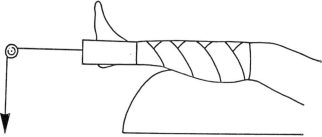

Fig. 4.5   Simple traction with the leg on a pillow and a pulley over the end of the bed.

Fig. 4.6(a)   Subcapital fracture of the neck of the femur; and **(b)** after replacement of the head with an Austin Moore prosthesis.

Fig. 4.4   Types of fracture of the neck of the femur according to the anatomical area. The stippled area is the neck and the striped area is the trochanteric region.

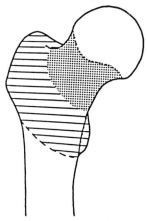

Initial management

It is important that these patients have their fractures dealt with expeditiously, and in some hospitals they have the fracture operated on as soon as they are assessed and an operating theatre is available. Most orthopaedic surgeons find that if the

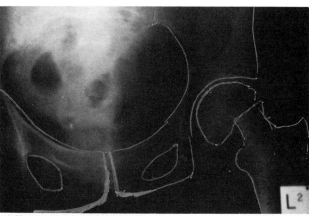

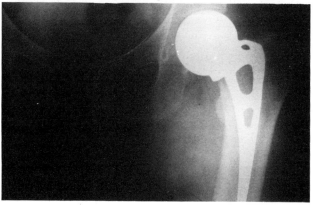

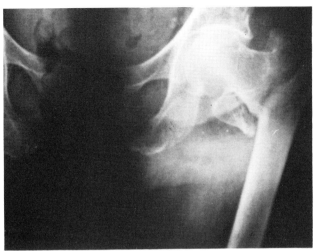

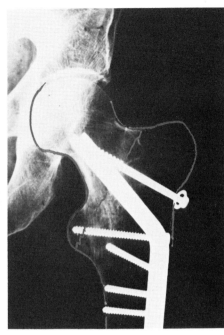

Fig. 4.7(a)   Pertrochanteric fracture of the neck of the femur; and (**b**) treatment by angle plate and lag screw.

Figures 4.6 and 4.7 show two types of fractured neck of the femur and the operations necessary.

Figures 4.8 to 4.10 show different internal fixation devices and differing techniques.

Fig. 4.8   Sliding screw for fractures of the neck of the femur.

Fig. 4.9   Angle plate and screws for subtrochanteric fracture of the femur.

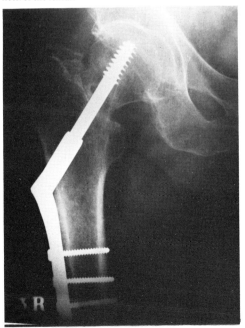

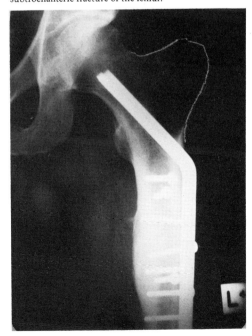

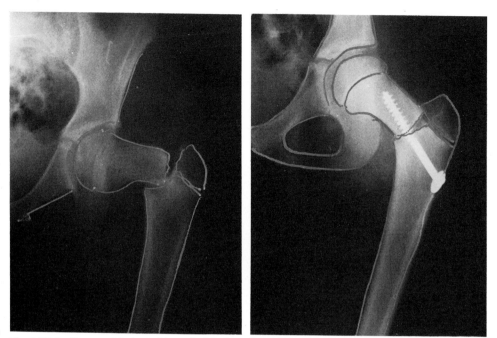

Fig. 4.10(a) Fracture of the base of the neck of the femur in a child; and **(b)** excellent reduction and fixation with a screw.

Other femoral fractures

General remarks − adults and children

All parts of the femur may be fractured − see Figure 4.11:

Nos. 1 and 2 − Neck and trochanteric region fractures have already been dealt with above.

No. 3 − Shaft fracture of femur.

No. 4 − Supracondylar fracture of femur.

No. 5 − Condylar fracture of femur (or femoral condyles).

Fractures of the femur are quite common in children because the femur is comparatively weak, especially against twisting forces.

In adults (Fig. 4.12), the femoral shaft is strong and it takes a lot of force to break the bone. It may be an isolated injury but it is often

Fig. 4.11 A map of femoral fractures:

1=neck;
2=trochanteric;
3=shaft;
4=supracondylar;
5=femoral condyles.

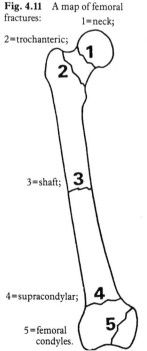

Fig. 4.12 Displaced fracture of the femoral shaft in an adult.

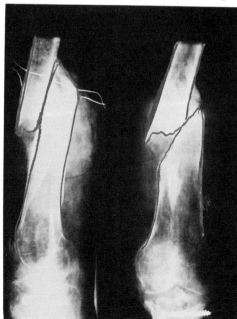

combined with other fractures and injuries, such as a head injury.

Even on its own, a fracture of the shaft of the femur causes shock from both pain and often blood loss into the thigh. This has been found to be several litres in some cases.

Initial management

1. Examine the patient carefully for other injuries.

2. Set up an intravenous drip and send blood for crossmatching, if the patient is clinically shocked.

3. Arrange X-rays and keep the leg splinted during this time.

Compound fractures (Figs. 4.13 and 4.14)

These need special care – see Chapter 1.

After the patient has been X-rayed you will need to arrange admission.

Operative treatment may be undertaken immediately, or after a few days, depending on the fracture and other injuries.

Conservative management is not used as frequently as in the past, because the results of operative treatment have continued to improve with better techniques.

You will need to know how to set up a fractured femur: in both skin traction, for temporary traction prior to an operation; and skeletal traction, when traction is to be the treatment of choice.

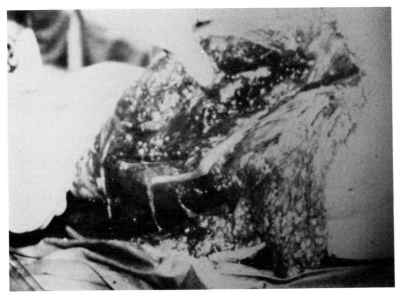

Fig. 4.13   A huge compound wound over the shaft of the femur.

Fig. 4.14   The X-rays of the patient shown in Fig. 4.13, showing a comminuted fracture of shaft of the femur.

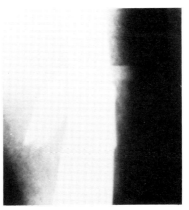
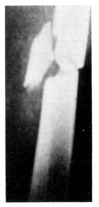

How to set up traction (Hamilton Russell type)

If the patient is in pain, insert a femoral nerve block before handling the fractured leg (see last section of Chapter 1).

Use a prepared skin traction kit, if available, otherwise use non-stretch, non-allergic tape. The leg should be shaved down each side and Tincture of Benzoin applied. The traction strip is then bandaged on (see Fig. 4.15). **It is important that the strip does not extend to the knee on the lateral side, as traction over the head of the fibula can damage the peroneal nerve.**

A wide sling is then put under the knee with suitable padding in the sling. A rope then goes to an overhead pulley and down to a bar on the traction frame at the foot of the bed, then to the spreader block, back to the frame pulley and down

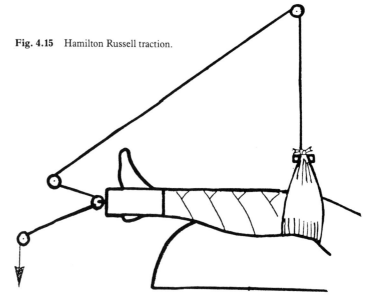

Fig. 4.15   Hamilton Russell traction.

to the weight (see Fig. 4.16). You will need about 4kg in the weight bag. A soft pillow goes under the calf, but the heel should be free from pressure.

Fig. 4.16   A patient with a fractured femur in Hamilton Russell traction.

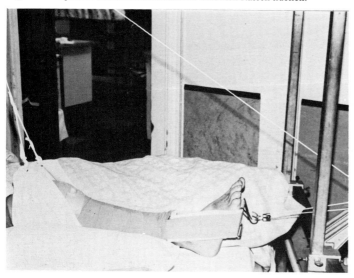

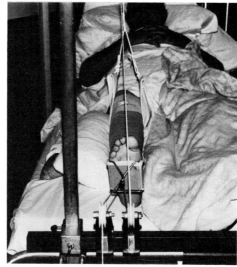

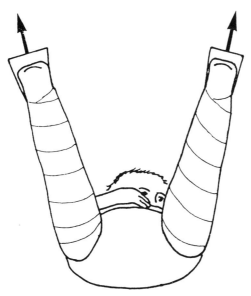

Fig. 4.17 Gallows traction.

Fig. 4.18 Gallows traction – the position of the feet.

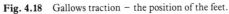

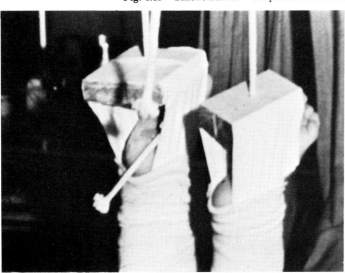

Skin traction – Gallows traction

This type of traction (Fig. 4.17) is used for fractures of the femur in young children up to the age of two years, or slightly older, depending on the size of the child.

Traction is applied after suitable analgesics have been given. Two lots of skin traction are applied (one to each leg) and the ropes are then applied to an overhead pulley system.

The legs should be slightly externally rotated and abducted (Fig. 4.18). The weights necessary are roughly 12.5 per cent of the weight of the child (on each leg). It should *just* lift the child's bottom off of the mattress.

The knees should be kept slightly flexed in the older child; and a splint is necessary to hold them in this position and prevent too much pulling on the femoral artery against the inguinal ligament. This is the danger in the older, larger child.

Skeletal traction

This may be used as the definitive
treatment, with or without an
attempt at closed reduction (Fig.
4.19).

It may also be used to keep a
fracture from shortening whilst you
await the opportunity to carry out
internal fixation (Figs. 4.19 and
4.20).

Whether a modified Thomas
splint is used or not, you will need
to know how to insert the tibial pin
to set up skeletal traction. If a
Thomas splint is used, choose one
that has a diameter about five
centimetres bigger than the
circumference of the thigh. Use
flannelette or towelling across the
splint and a large pad under the
fracture site. The splint, when in
place, should push up against the
ischial tuberosity.

Even if you have inserted a
femoral nerve block, you will need
to supplement this with some local
anaesthetic at the site of insertion of
the pin and on the opposite side of
the tibia where the pin comes out.

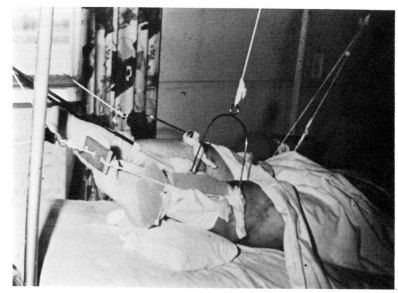

Fig. 4.19 Bilateral skeletal traction – with one leg in a Thomas splint and the other in a
modified skeletal Hamilton Russell traction. The patient weighed 180kg.

Fig. 4.20 Simple skeletal traction to maintain length in a fractured femur preoperatively.

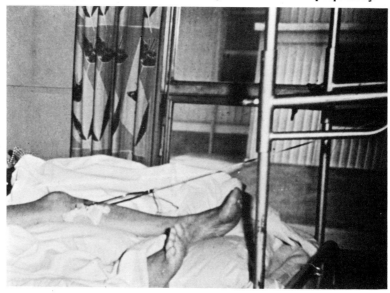

The pin is inserted 2cm posterior to the tibial tuberosity and parallel to the mattress or the floor (Fig. 4.21).

It is best to use a threaded pin, such as Denham pin, and in order to avoid heat damage to the bone, the hole should be drilled with an appropriately sized bit at a slow speed. Tap the hole and thereby cut the thread.

Whilst this is being done, you will need help to steady the leg and to advise you if you are drilling the hole in the correct alignment. When all this has been done, balance the weight of the splint, as shown in Figure 4.22, and apply enough weight to maintain the alignment.

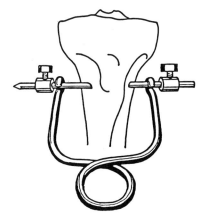

Fig. 4.21 The site of insertion of skeletal traction in the upper tibia.

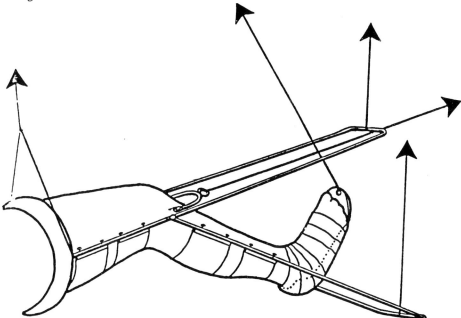

Fig. 4.22 Balanced skeletal traction in a Thomas splint with a Pearson knee flexion device.

Supracondylar fractures

Undisplaced fractures of the supracondylar region may be treated with an initial period of bed rest in simple traction or a light plaster. This can be followed by mobilization in a cast-brace or caliper.

Displaced fractures (Fig. 4.23) give poor results with conservative management, therefore they usually require open reduction (Fig. 4.24) as re-alignment by closed means is seldom satisfactory.

Beware of damage to femoral vessels. Check the circulation in the leg and if damaged, **urgent** repair is necessary.

Traction is needed, whilst awaiting an operation (see the preceding section for details). Traction is set up after a femoral nerve block has been inserted into the femoral nerve, just below the inguinal ligament (see last section of Chapter 1 for details).

Some examples of these fractures and their appropriate internal fixation are shown in Figures 4.24, 4.25 and 4.26.

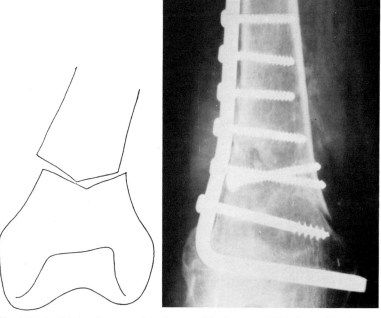

Fig. 4.23(a)   Displaced supracondylar fracture of the femur; and **(b)** its internal fixation.

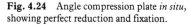

Fig. 4.24   Angle compression plate *in situ*, showing perfect reduction and fixation.

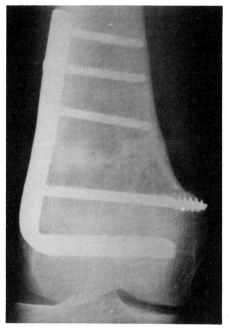

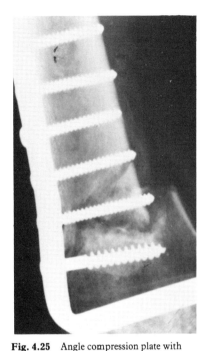

Fig. 4.25 Angle compression plate with some acceptable displacement.

Fig. 4.26 Plate and screw fixation of supracondylar fracture.

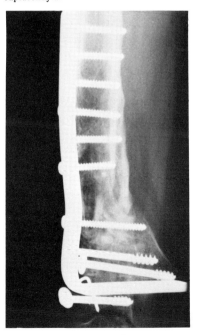

Femoral condyles

These are intra-articular fractures (Fig. 4.27) and the future function of the joint depends on the early and accurate reduction and fixation of this fracture.

Prior to the operation, the patient should rest in bed in a long leg backslab with the knee slightly flexed. The backslab needs to be well padded.

Figure 4.28 is an example of operative repair using multiple lag screws.

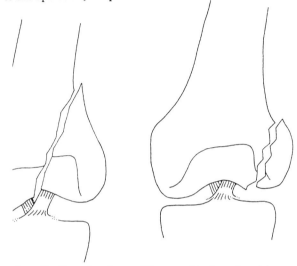

Fig. 4.27 Examples of types of fractures of the femoral condyles.

Fig. 4.28 Screw fixation for fractures of the femoral condyles.

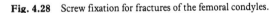

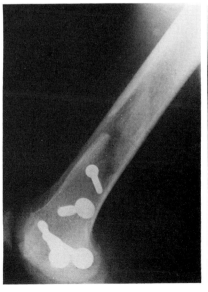

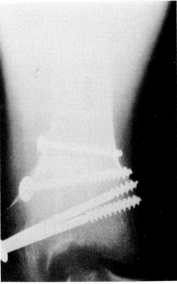

Fractures of the patella

Patella fractures are commonly the result of:

1. A direct blow on the kneecap. These fractures are often comminuted, and can be compound (Fig. 4.29).

2. Muscular action – caused by sudden contraction of the quadriceps. These fractures are transverse, not comminuted and rarely compound (Fig. 4.30).

If the fracture is undisplaced (Figs. 4.31 and 4.32), then a long leg, padded, backslab plaster or cylinder needs to be applied. Crutches will be necessary for a few days, then weight can be taken on the leg (Fig. 4.33).

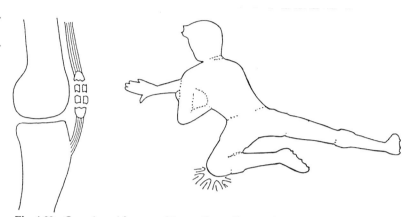

Fig. 4.29   Comminuted fractures of the patella usually result from a direct blow.

Fig. 4.30   Transverse fractures of the patella are usually the result of muscular action.

Fig. 4.31   Undisplaced and incomplete fracture of the patella.

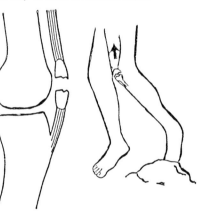 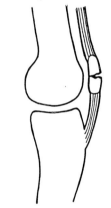

Fig. 4.32   Lateral X-ray of a fracture of the lower pole of the patella.

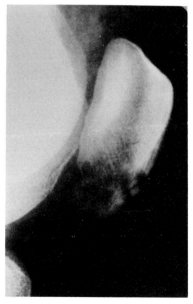

In these cases, the quadriceps mechanism is intact and the plaster simply protects the injured part of the mechanism from splitting apart by preventing knee flexion. The slab can be completed to form a cylinder, after the swelling goes down (see next section for details) and will need to be kept on for four to six weeks, as a rule.

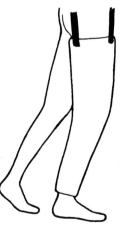

Fig. 4.33   Mobilization in a plaster cylinder with weight bearing.

Application of a plaster slab

A long leg plaster slab is often used in the management of a fractured patella.

To apply this, you will need a plaster slab that extends from 5cm above the ankle to the upper third of the thigh. The slab should be of eighteen layers of plaster bandage.

First, apply a length of stockingette over the leg, leaving extra length at the proximal and distal ends. Then put a circle of felt around the distal and proximal part of the leg and thigh respectively exactly where the slab will end (Fig. 4.34). Apply a generous layer of Velband, Webril or rolled wool and then apply the slab posteriorly. Now bandage it onto the leg with a firm crepe bandage. Turn back the spare stockingette over the ring of felt and bandage it onto the slab and the leg, so that each end is padded (Fig. 4.34).

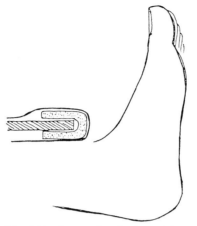

Fig. 4.34   Cross section of a plaster slab or cylinder showing the padding at either end.

Plaster cylinder

Use the same technique as above, only the slab needs to be only twelve layers and instead of using a crepe bandage to hold the slab on, you use 15cm plaster bandages (Fig. 4.35).

A plaster cylinder (Fig. 4.33) is heavy and when you stand up it will slide down the leg, become loose, and press on the tendo-achilles. To avoid this, when the plaster is dry, you can drill a hole through the plaster near the proximal end (anteriorly and posteriorly) and thread a tape through the holes. This can then be tied to a belt around the waist.

Fig. 4.35   Plaster cylinder.

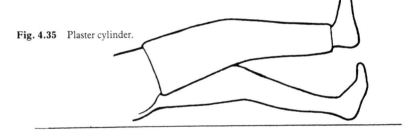

Displaced fractures

Here the extensor mechanism has been ruptured and the patient finds that he or she is unable to lift the leg with the knee out straight (Fig. 4.36).

A similar problem exists when the quadriceps muscle is ruptured, or the patellar tendon is ruptured (Fig. 4.37).

In all these cases, repair of the quadriceps mechanism is essential.

Apply a padded, long leg, backslab and arrange the operation.

Patellar fractures are treated by tension band wiring (Figs. 4.38 and 4.39). Compound fractures are treated as outlined in Chapter 1.

Some surgeons treat comminuted fractures of the patella by excision of the patella. I believe that the patella is important and try to preserve it in all patients.

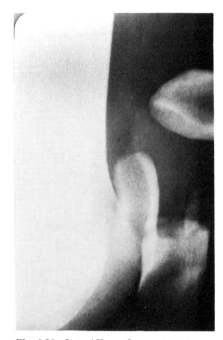

Fig. 4.36   Lateral X-ray of a comminuted fracture of the patella – there is disruption of the extensor mechanism.

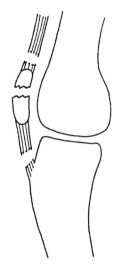

Fig. 4.37   Types of rupture of the quadriceps mechanism.

Fig. 4.38   Tension band wiring in antero-posterior X-ray of patella.

Fig. 4.39   Tension band wiring in lateral X-ray of patella.

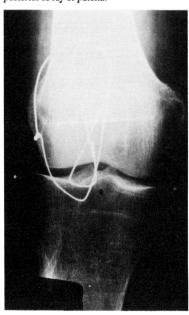

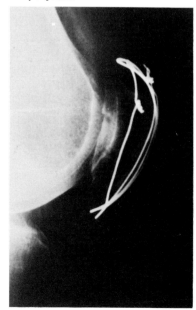

Fractures of the tibia

These are amongst the commonest of the fractures of long bones. The fractures occur in a variety of ways, from simple twisting injuries to severe high speed injuries with tissue damage.

Compound fractures are dealt with in Chapter 1.

As there are differences in treatment, fractures of the tibia will be dealt with in three sections (Fig. 4.40):

1. Fractures of the plateau region of the tibia;

2. Fractures of the shaft of the tibia; and

3. Fractures involving the ankle joint.

The plateau region

These fractures are often caused by a fall from a height and tend to occur in an older age group. There is often crushing of the cancellous bone of the upper tibia (Fig. 4.41).

Minor degrees of depression (Fig. 4.41) require immobilization in a long leg plaster – but remember that this is an intra-articular fracture, so it is important that treatment should try to reconstruct the joint surface, if it is significantly depressed (Fig. 4.42). There are three ways of doing this:

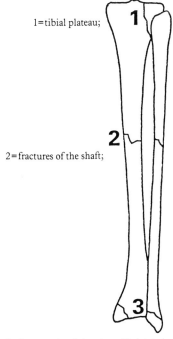

Fig. 4.40 Sites of fractures of the tibia:

1=tibial plateau;

2=fractures of the shaft;

3=fractures involving the ankle joint.

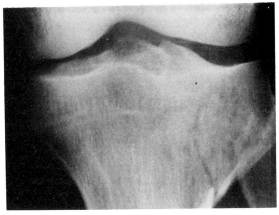

Fig. 4.41 Fracture of the lateral tibial plateau with little displacement or depression of the articular surface.

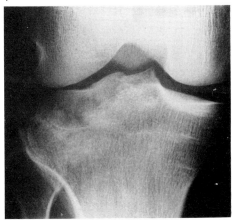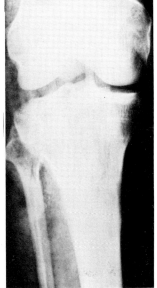

Fig. 4.42(a) Significant depression and disruption of the articular surface of the lateral tibial plateau; **(b)** well reduced and in plaster.

1. By closed reduction (if possible) and plaster, followed by intensive physiotherapy for four to six months.

Initially put the patient in a backslab. Reduction will need to be under a general anaesthetic.

Compression of the fragments (Fig. 4.43) and moulding are necessary. A well moulded plaster needs to be applied.

2. By traction and early active exercises against the pull of the traction (Fig. 4.44). Skeletal traction is inserted a little lower down the shaft of the tibia than usual (Fig. 4.21).

A Denham pin, which differs from a Steinman pin by being threaded, is best (see earlier section on *Skeletal traction* in this chapter). The patient stays in hospital.

Traction is kept on for three weeks with increasing exercise. Crutches

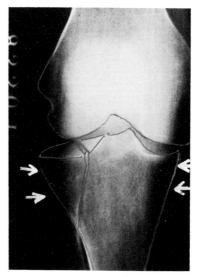

Fig. 4.43   Closed reduction, needs compression of the fragments if possible.

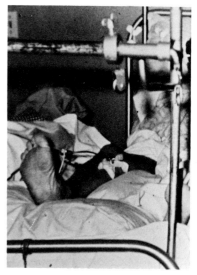

Fig. 4.44   Traction through a Denham pin, a little lower than usual.

will be needed for a further three to four weeks and then limited activity is allowed.

3. By operation (Figs. 4.45 and 4.46). This has the advantage of: accurate reduction; a short stay in hospital; and early restoration of function, without plaster.

Fig. 4.45   Severe disruption of tibial plateau – almost a dislocated knee.

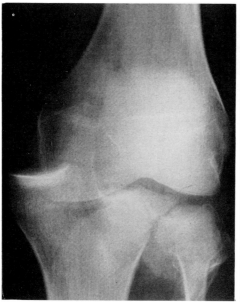
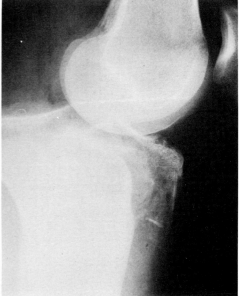

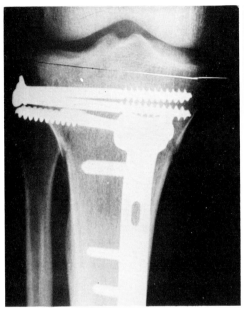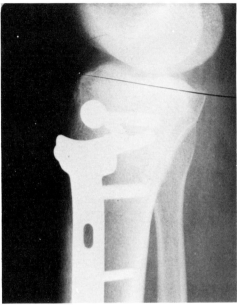

Fig. 4.46 The same case as in Figure 4.45 after reduction and internal fixation.

Some examples are shown in Figs. 4.47 and 4.48.

Before the operation, immobilize the patient in a long leg, padded, slab.

Fig. 4.48 Compression screw, K-wire, buttress plate and bone graft were used in this excellent reconstruction.

Fig. 4.47 Compression screws for reconstruction of the plateau.

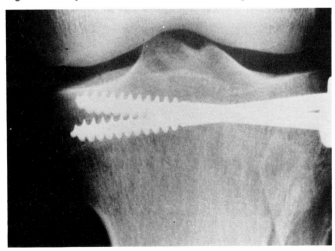

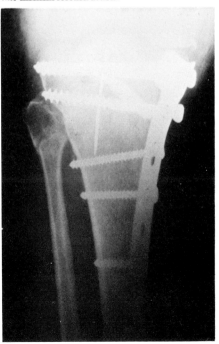

The shaft

There are three basic types of fracture:

1. Simple – often caused by sport, such as skiing and soccer, or a motor vehicle accident (Fig. 4.49).

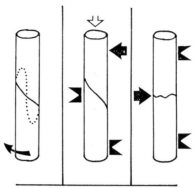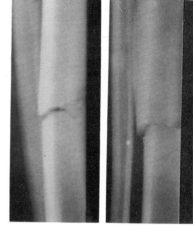

Fig. 4.49   Simple fractures of the tibia and the forces causing them.

2. Butterfly – the 'bumper bar' fracture, or from a heavy fall while skiing (Fig. 4.50).

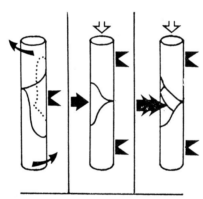

Fig. 4.50   Butterfly fractures of the tibia and the forces causing them.

3. Comminuted – caused by high speed motor accidents, skiing and crush injuries (Fig. 4.51).

Each of these basic types of fracture of the tibia can be: undisplaced or displaced; and closed or open (compound).

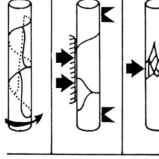

Fig. 4.51   Comminuted fractures of the tibia and the forces causing them.

Undisplaced fractures of the tibia and fibula

These require immobilization in a long leg plaster with the knee flexed 10 to 15 degrees and the ankle at 90 degrees (Fig. 4.52).

The following technique is a good way to apply the plaster and control the fracture.

The plaster is put on in two sections: The first, is put on below the knee. With the surgeon seated, the padding is applied by an assistant while the surgeon controls and protects the fracture (Fig. 4.53).

When the first section is firm, the top half of the plaster can be applied (Fig. 4.54).

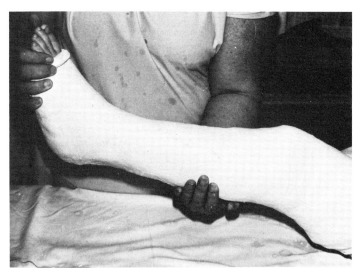

Fig. 4.52   A padded, long leg, plaster which should extend from the upper thigh to the metatarsal heads.

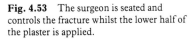

Fig. 4.53   The surgeon is seated and controls the fracture whilst the lower half of the plaster is applied.

Fig. 4.54   With the lower half of the plaster applied and the fracture controlled, the upper part can be applied − note the padding.

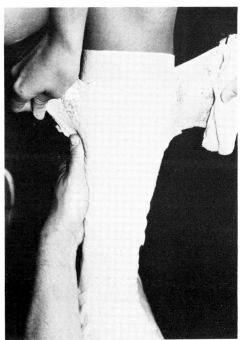

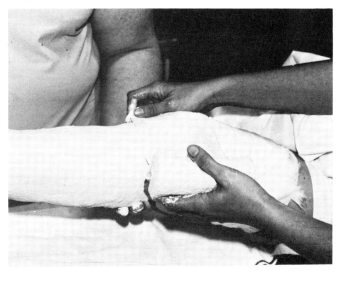

Another way is for a second assistant to support the leg at the fracture site and under the thigh whilst the surgeon controls the leg by both traction and direct pressure and later by moulding as the plaster sets (Fig. 4.55). He should stand at the foot of the table and the patient should be pulled down so that the sole of the patient's foot rests on his abdomen.

In a recent fracture, where swelling is to be expected, the plaster should be well padded and the patient kept in hospital − so that the circulation in the toes can be checked.

If there is any doubt about the plaster being too tight, the whole length of the plaster is split to the skin (using a plaster saw and a spreader to slightly open the plaster) so that the leg is left in a shell.

A long leg plaster extends from the metatarsal heads to the upper third of the thigh. Special attention needs to be paid to padding the heel, the malleoli and the knee region over the head of the fibula.

Undisplaced fractures of the tibia and fibula shafts need six to eight weeks in a child to unite (Fig. 4.56) and 14 to 16 weeks in an adult. It will take many months to regain knee and ankle movements and agility.

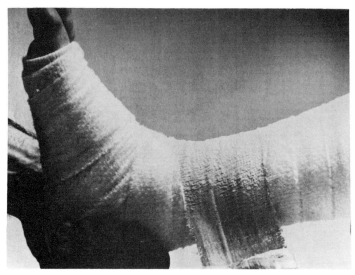

Fig. 4.55   Another method. The surgeon stands at the end of the table, controls the fracture and pulls on the leg, whilst the plaster is applied.

Fig. 4.56   Spiral fracture of the middle third of the tibia in good position in plaster.

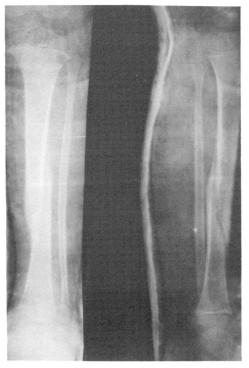

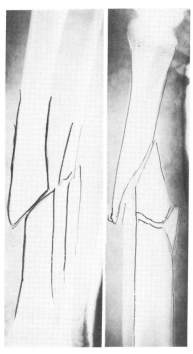

Displaced fractures of the tibia and fibula

Displacement and shortening (Fig. 4.57a) or angulation (Fig. 4.57b) cannot be accepted in this day and age, so the displaced fracture requires reduction.

Reduction can be either closed or open.

Closed reduction

Displaced and angulated fractures will need to be reduced under a general anaesthetic with a combination of traction and direct pressure (Fig. 4.58).

Is reduction acceptable? Take an X-ray after reduction and if the reduction is not yet satisfactory, a further attempt may be made.

Fig. 4.58 Closed reduction of fractures of the tibia and fibula by traction and direct pressure.

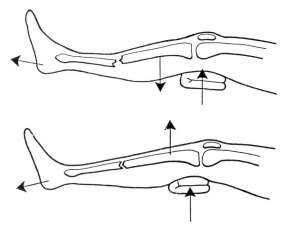

Fig. 4.57(a) Butterfly fracture of the tibia and fibula with shortening. **(b)** transverse fracture of the tibia and fibula with gross angulation.

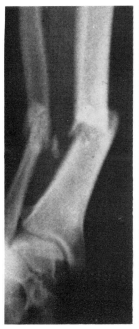

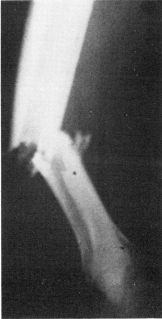

Reduction is acceptable if:
1. There is no shortening;
2. There is no angulation; or
3. There is 50 per cent or more apposition.

Figure 4.59 shows a fracture in an acceptable position, whilst Figure 4.60 is unacceptable.

Angulation and some malrotation can be corrected (Fig. 4.61) by wedging the plaster.

All displaced fractures should be put in well padded plasters when reduced and the plaster should be then split to allow for swelling.

The patient should stay in hospital for 24 hours and the plaster can then be completed if there is no undue swelling, and the patient mobilized. Most patients have **a lot of pain in the first few days and require analgesics.**

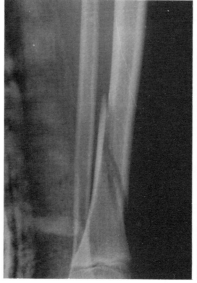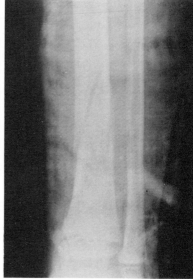

Fig. 4.59   Acceptable position of the fracture.

Fig. 4.60   Unacceptable position.

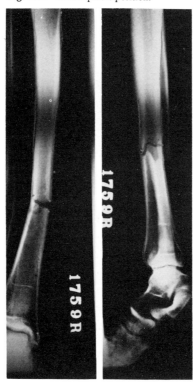

Fig. 4.61   Site of wedge to be opened, and rotation to be corrected.

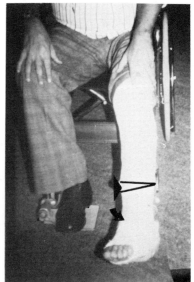

Open reduction and internal fixation

Open reduction and internal fixation is now commonly used. The decision to carry out open reduction and internal fixation is one that will be made by the orthopaedic surgeon, based on his approach to the problem posed by the various types of fractures of the tibia.

You must supply an accurate description of the fracture and, if the patient is to have a delayed operation, immobilize the fracture in a long leg, padded, backslab that adequately holds the fracture and controls pain.

Some examples of some of the different techniques are shown in Figs. 4.62 to 4.65.

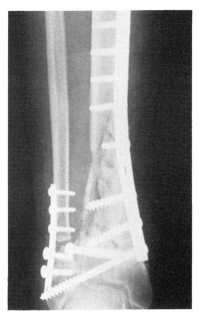

Fig. 4.62 Severely comminuted fracture of the tibia and fibula treated by open reduction and internal fixation.

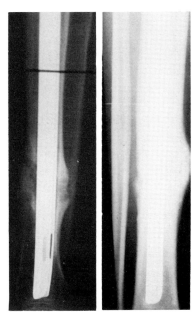

Fig. 4.63 Medullary nailing of a fractured tibia and fibula.

Fig. 4.64 Compression plating for a short oblique fracture of the tibia and fibula.

Fig. 4.65 Some compression techniques.

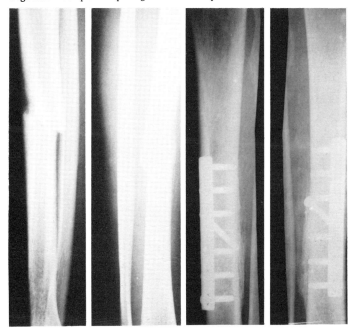

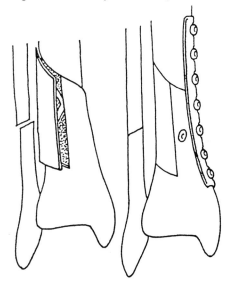

Compound fractures of the tibia and fibula (Figs. 4.66 and 4.67)

These have been dealt with in Chapter 1, as far as the wound is concerned. The fracture itself can then be treated in a number of ways following debridement of the wound:

1. Closed reduction and a long leg plaster;
2. Internal fixation; and
3. External fixation.

External fixation (Fig. 4.68) allows for immobilization of the fracture, and also allows access to the wound and mobility of the joints. It is now frequently used.

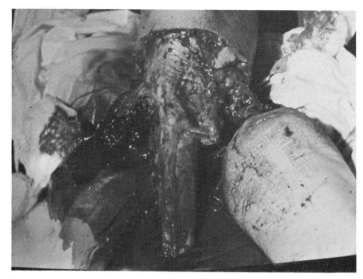

Fig. 4.66 Horrendous compound wound.

Fig. 4.67 The X-rays of wound shown in Figure 4.66.

Fig. 4.68 *Fixateur Externe* in place on a fractured tibia and fibula.

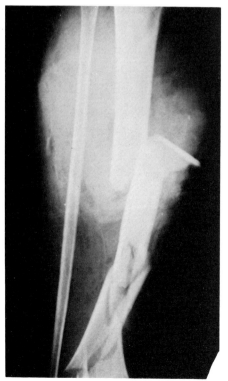

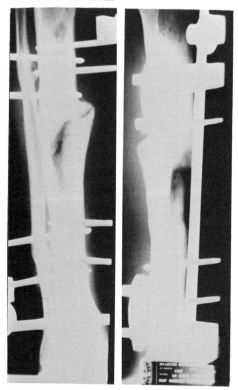

Fractures of the fibula

These fractures can be:

1. Associated with fractures of the tibia (Fig. 4.69), in which case, the treatment is usually secondary to that of the major injury, the fractured tibia.

The latter will be treated in plaster or by open reduction and internal fixation. The fibula will heal as the tibia stabilizes.

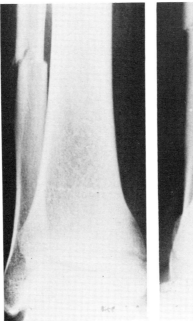
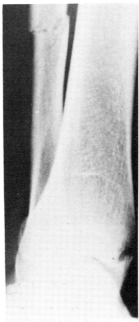

Fig. 4.70 Fracture of the fibula, in its middle third, associated with an ankle fracture.

Fig. 4.69 Fracture of the fibula. N.B. There is also a major fracture of the tibia.

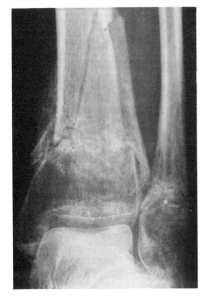

2. Associated with the ankle joint (Fig. 4.70) see the next section on *Fractures of the distal tibia and fibula involving the ankle joint.*

3. Isolated fractures (Fig. 4.71). These are usually caused by direct injury to the fibula.

Beware! A high spiral fracture of the fibula may be associated with an ankle injury.

Fig. 4.71 Isolated fracture of the fibula.

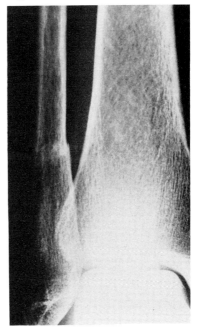

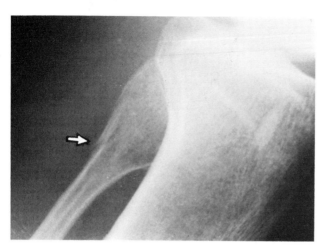

Fig. 4.72   Fracture of the neck of the fibula.

Displacement is rare. Local tenderness, if severe, may justify a short leg walking plaster (see *How to apply a short leg walking plaster* – in the next section).

Usually, a crepe bandage or elastic stocking and restricted activity for 3 weeks is all that is necessary.

Fractures of the head and neck of the fibula (Fig. 4.72) may damage the lateral popliteal nerve and thus cause foot drop.

Fractures of the ankle

The distal tibia and fibula involving the ankle joint

The name **'Pott's fracture'** is always associated with almost all ankle fractures and yet Percival Pott (1714-1788) – who was said to have suffered such a fracture when thrown from a horse in 1756 – probably simply had a compound fracture of the tibia and fibula, and not an ankle fracture at all.

Pott's disease (tuberculosis of the spine) is also named after him.

If Percival Pott did not have his own fracture, then what is a Pott's fracture? It has become a general name for all fractures and fracture dislocations of the ankle.

Look at the Figures 4.73 to 4.76.

Are they all Pott's fractures?

Yes, they are.

How can you accurately and quickly understand what has happened to the ankle and describe the injury?

Fig. 4.73   An example of a Pott's fracture of the ankle.

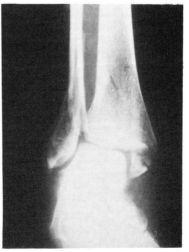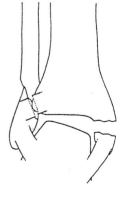

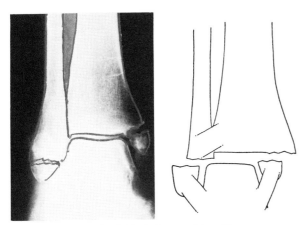

Fig. 4.74   An example of a Pott's fracture of the ankle.

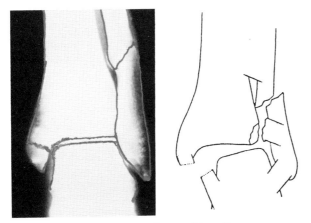

Fig. 4.75   An example of a Pott's fracture of the ankle.

Fig. 4.76   An example of a Pott's fracture of the ankle.

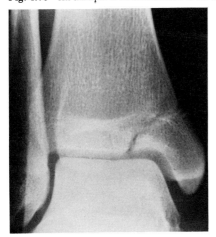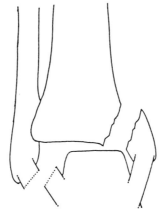

Let me introduce the *circle concept*.
Study the circle I have drawn on
Figures 4.77 and 4.78. Follow the
circle and comment on the
following:

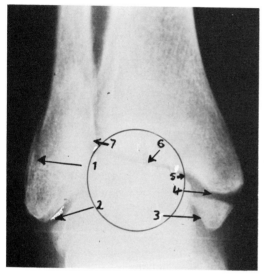

Antero-posterior view (Fig. 4.77)

1. Lateral malleolus − spiral fracture
2. Lateral ligament − intact
3. Medial ligament − intact
4. Medial malleolus − transverse displaced fracture
5. Articular surface of tibia − intact
6. Articular surface of talus − intact
7. Tibio-fibular ligament − intact

Fig. 4.77   The circle concept − Antero-posterior view.

Fig. 4.78   The circle concept − Lateral view.

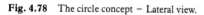

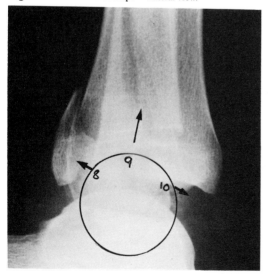

Lateral view (Fig. 4.78)

8. Posterior articular surface − small fragment
9. Lateral view of spiral fracture of lateral malleolus
10. Anterior capsule ligaments − ruptured.

Now try the system on Figures

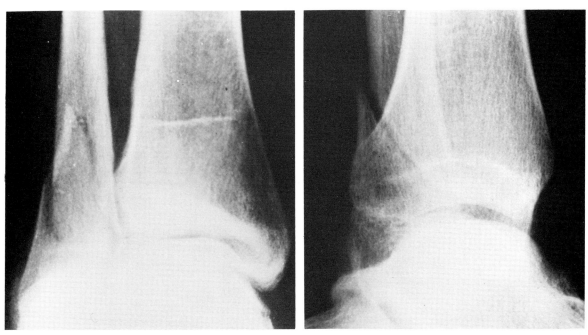

Fig. 4.79 Test fracture for the circle concept.

Fig. 4.80 Test fracture for the circle concept.

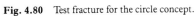

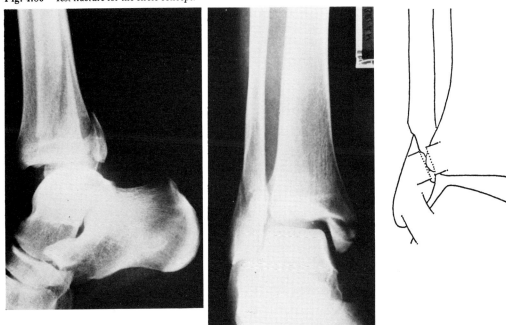

Answers:

Figure 4.79. Spiral fracture of lateral malleolus but all other structures intact. Therefore no displacement.

Figure 4.80. Spiral fracture of lateral malleolus; horizontal avulsion fracture of medial malleolus below joint line; one third of the posterior articular surface is fractured and displaced proximally; and the anterior capsule is ruptured. This is a *Type A* fracture (see below) with displacement.

 In addition to a description of the fracture, a classification system is necessary.

How can we classify such a group of fractures?

The key is the tibio-fibular ligament (the syndesmotic ligament, which has an anterior and a posterior element).

Type A (Figs. 4.81 and 4.82)

Tibio-fibular ligament intact.

 Fracture of lateral malleolus, at or below the joint line.

 Medial malleolus may be fractured, or medial ligament ruptured.

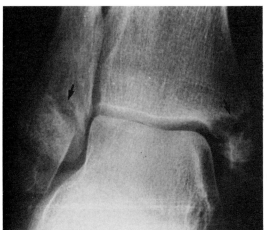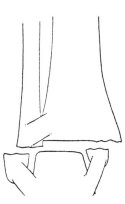

Fig. 4.81   Type A fracture.

Fig. 4.82   Type A fracture.

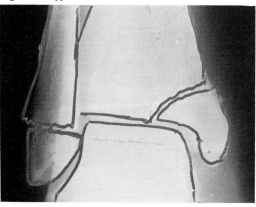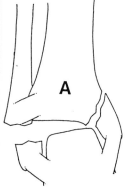

Type B (Figs. 4.83 and 4.84)

Tibio-fibular ligament partially ruptured.

  Fracture at level of ankle spirals proximally.

  There may be a piece off the lateral side of the tibia.

  Medial malleolus is avulsed, or the medial ligament ruptured.

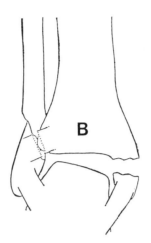
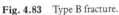

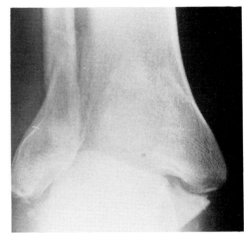

Fig. 4.83   Type B fracture.   **Fig. 4.84**   Type C fracture.

Type C (Fig. 4.85a and b)

Tibio-fibular ligament completely ruptured.

  Fracture of the lateral malleolus above the ankle joint.

  Syndesmosis (tibiofibular ligament) is ruptured – often a piece of tibia is pulled off with it.

  Medial malleolus is avulsed, or the medial ligament ruptured.

Fig. 4.85   Type C fracture.

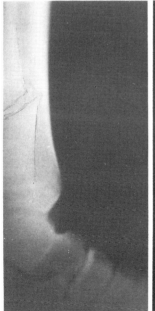
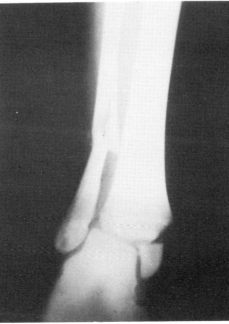
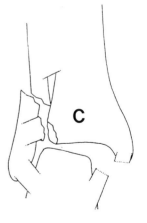

Fig. 4.86 X-rays of a Type B fracture.

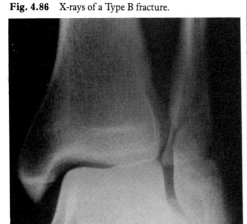

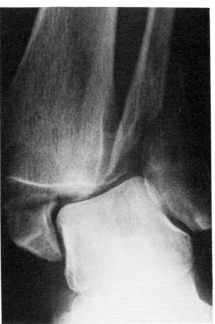

Management

Some ankle fractures are markedly displaced and therefore there is pressure on the skin. If you see such a fracture, a quick pull on the foot will partly reduce the fracture and ease the pressure on the skin, which can quickly become necrotic.

Reduction of the fracture can be either closed or open.

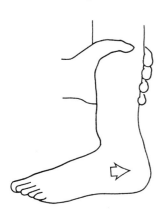

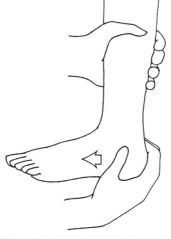

Fig. 4.87 Correct the posterior shift by lifting the heel forward.

Closed reduction

This must be perfect or it is unacceptable. Also perfect positioning must be maintained, even after the swelling has gone down.

Unless reduction is perfect and the fracture remains undisplaced, re-reduction or open reduction and internal fixation are necessary.

Many surgeons (including myself) regard open reduction and internal fixation as the treatment of choice for displaced ankle fractures.

Let's look at the reduction of a Type B fracture (Fig. 4.86 – the most common one) with lateral or posterior displacement.

Firstly, correct the posterior shift by lifting the heel forward (Fig. 4.87); then the lateral displacement is corrected by firm pressure (Fig. 4.88) – note the position of the hands (Fig. 4.89).

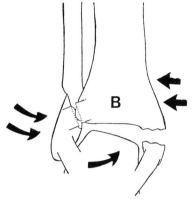

Fig. 4.88   Correct the lateral displacement with direct pressure (Type B fracture).

Fig. 4.89   Note the position of the hands during reduction of the lateral shift.

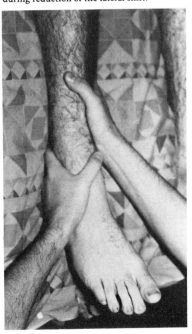

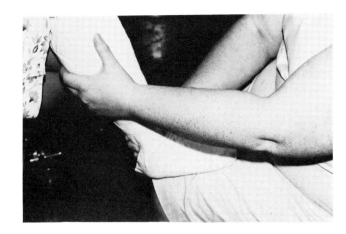

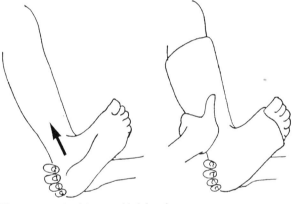

Fig. 4.90(a)   Applying a padded short leg plaster.
(b)   Diagram to show how the foot is held and the plaster moulded.

When you have obtained reduction – there is a definite end point – maintain it. Apply a well padded plaster with moulding (Fig. 4.90a and b).

In line with our earlier advice, the plaster should be split (Fig. 4.91) to allow for swelling. (Remember – No recent fracture has a complete plaster left enclosing the limb.)

Fig. 4.91   Split the plaster down to the skin in a recent fracture.

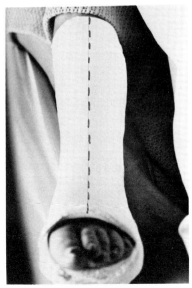

Closed reduction of a Type A fracture

Where the displacement of the talus and the foot is to the lateral side the pressure will be as before . . . over the lateral malleolus with counter pressure above the medial malleolus (Fig. 4.92a).

The hands will be reversed from their position above if it is a vertical fracture of the medial malleolus with medial displacement of the talus and foot and the pressure will be from the medial side with counter pressure above the lateral malleolus.

Closed reduction of a Type C fracture

You need a lot of direct pressure over the lateral side and counter pressure medially.
Do not try to squeeze the fracture together (Fig. 4.94a), as you will be unsuccessful. . . . The counter-pressure hand should always be more proximal.

How to apply a short leg plaster

First make a backslab which extends from the metatarsal heads to 4cm below the knee. This must consist of 12 layers of plaster, 15cm wide.

Apply padding, especially over the malleoli and the heel (Fig. 4.93).

Unless you are an expert, you will need an assistant to hold the foot at 90 degrees, either by holding the toes or use the stockingette to hold the leg at an angle of 90 (Fig. 4.93).

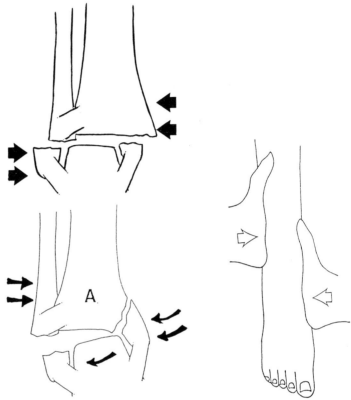

Fig. 4.92(a)   Reduction of Type A fracture with lateral displacement.
(b)   Type A fracture with medial displacement.
(c)   Reduction of fracture in **(b)**.

Fig. 4.93   Application of a short leg plaster – apply the padding and keep the ankle at 90 degrees.

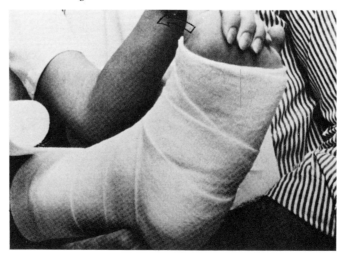

Apply two circular 15cm plaster bandages, starting at the toes and moving up half a width of the bandage every second turn. The proximal level is 3cm below the neck of the fibula.

Note that the moulding is done with the hands at different levels (Fig. 4.94b). Moulding by squeezing or with the hands at the wrong levels (Fig. 4.94a) is not effective, and the fracture will not be reduced.

Mould the fracture and hold until set.

Apply the slab and bandage with a 15cm circular plaster bandage, after turning back the excess stockingette.

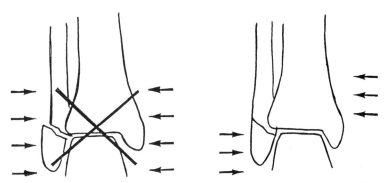

Fig. 4.94 The futility of squeezing the fracture, instead of moulding the fracture and the plaster.

A heel is applied only in undisplaced Type A fractures – an extra slab of ten thicknesses is applied to the sole, the heel is placed in the centre of the sole and bandaged onto the plaster with a 10cm plaster bandage (Fig. 4.96).

You will need a post-reduction X-ray.

Fig. 4.95 The hands are at the wrong level for moulding this plaster.

Fig. 4.96 A short leg plaster with a walking heel.

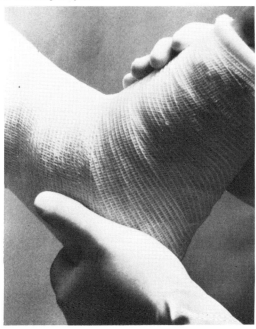

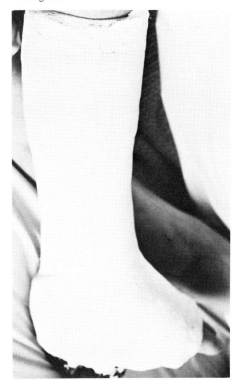

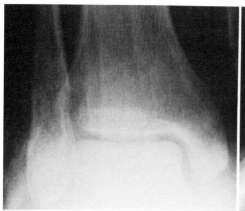

Fig. 4.97   Good reduction of an ankle fracture.

Fig. 4.98   The criterion of good reduction – equal joint space all the way round the ankle.

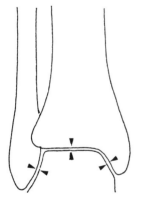

Fig. 4.99   Poor reduction – uneven joint space.

Is the fracture (Figs. 4.97 and 4.99) reduced satisfactorily?

Figure 4.97 shows good reduction – note that the joint space is even all the way around (Fig. 4.98).

Figure 4.99 shows poor reduction – the joint space is uneven.

The patient will need to stay in hospital for one or two days with the leg elevated on a pillow.

Open the split plaster (Fig. 4.100), if there is any doubt about it being too tight.

After 24 hours, provided there is no undue swelling, the plaster can be completed again. The patient can be mobilized on crutches and discharged home.

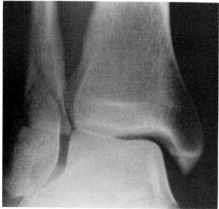

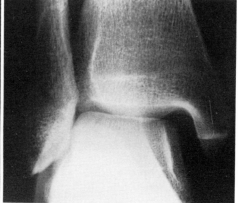

Removal of a short leg plaster

A reciprocating saw (Fig. 4.101) should be used, especially if a walking heel has been added, as the plaster is then very thick. The trouble with the saw is that it is noisy and frightens people, especially children. You must demonstrate to the patient that the saw does not cut skin by testing it on your own hand.

Plaster shears (Fig. 4.102) **should be used for children**, and can be used if you want some exercise for your biceps and pectoral muscles. I prefer to use the shears except for very thick plaster.

Cut along in the line of the dots shown (Fig. 4.102) going behind the malleoli and along each side of the leg plaster.

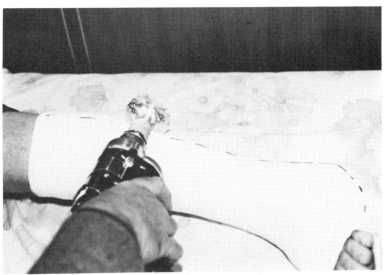

Fig. 4.101   The use of a reciprocating saw for plaster removal.

Fig. 4.102   Plaster shears for plaster removal from a child.

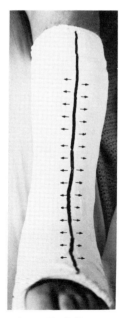

Fig. 4.100   Split and slightly open the plaster, if there is swelling and tightness.

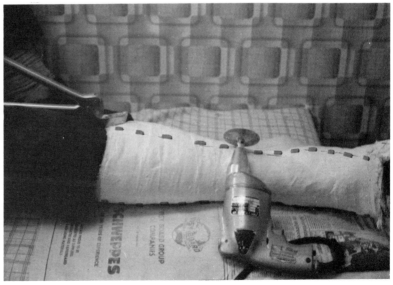

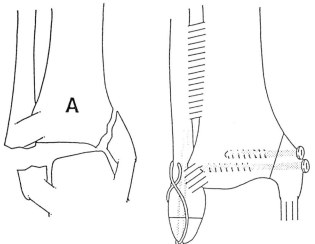

Fig. 4.103   Open reduction of a Type A fracture.

Fig. 4.104   Open reduction of a Type B fracture.

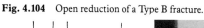

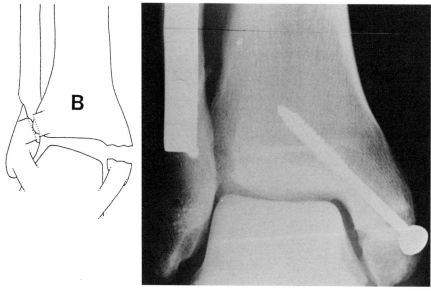

Open reduction of ankle fractures

Many surgeons (including myself) regard open reduction and internal fixation as the treatment of choice in displaced ankle fractures.

The reasons given include:
1. Perfect reduction
2. No plaster
3. Early mobilization
4. Rapid return of function
5. Better results.

Some examples of fixation techniques are shown in Figures 4.103 to 4.106.

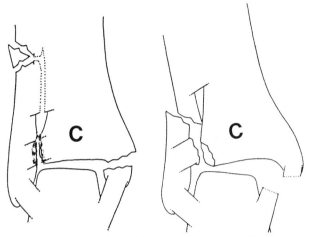

Whilst awaiting the operation, make sure that there is no pressure on the skin from bone fragments. Rest the patient in a short leg backslab.

Fig. 4.105   Two versions of a Type C fracture that need internal fixation.

Fig. 4.106   Internal fixation of a Type C fracture.

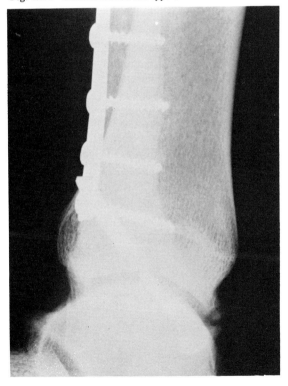

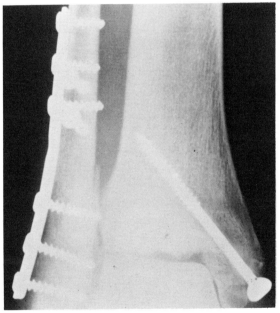

The talus

These fractures are not common and are often overlooked.

There are basically four bony injuries to the talus:

1. Fractures of the neck of the talus
2. Fractures of the dome of the talus
3. Fracture dislocations of the talus
4. Isolated fractures of the talus (posterior or lateral process).

1. *Fractures of the neck of the talus*
This fracture (Fig. 4.107) usually occurs as a result of forcible dorsiflexion of the ankle – the leading edge of the lower end of the tibia pushes into the narrow neck of the talus and it breaks.

Undisplaced fractures require immobilization in a short leg plaster for eight weeks, and then careful evaluation.

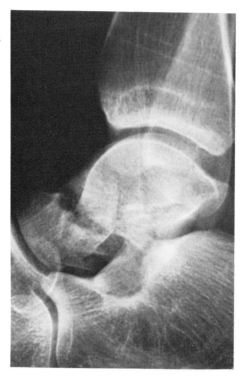

Fig. 4.107   Lateral X-ray of a fracture of the neck of the talus.

Be careful in saying the fracture is undisplaced because the distal fragment is often displaced dorsally (see Fig. 4.108) and as with all displaced fractures involving joints open reduction is advisable (see Fig. 4.109).

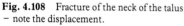

Fig. 4.108   Fracture of the neck of the talus – note the displacement.

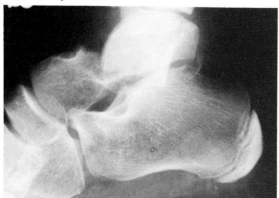

Fig. 4.109   The fracture shown in Figure 4.108 after open reduction and lag screw fixation.

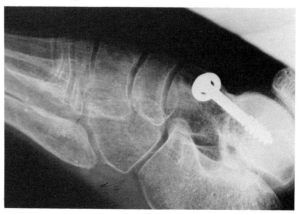

2. *Dome fractures of the talus*

In this case, a piece of the articular surface of the dorsal aspect of the talus (Fig. 4.110) is fractured and acts as a loose piece of bone.

The loose piece may require replacement and pinning, or removal and drilling of the bed from where the piece was avulsed.

3. *Fracture dislocation of the talus*

This is a serious and dramatic problem (Fig. 4.111). It is an extension of the fracture of the neck of the talus and arises from the same cause, namely a forced dorsiflexion injury associated with inversion.

The injury was common in air crashes. Now we see it more frequently in high speed motor vehicle accidents in small cars, in which the brake and clutch pedals are forcibly pushed against the foot.

The injury is often compound. See Chapter 1 for details of treatment of the compound wound.

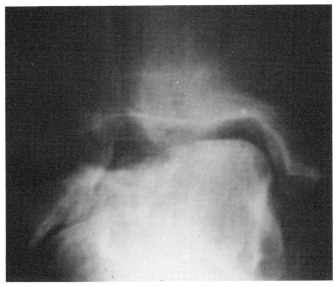

Fig. 4.110 Dome fracture of the talus — note the defect in the articular surface.

Even if there is no wound, the skin is often stretched very tightly and its chances of survival depend on rapid reduction.

Closed reduction is possible, but it is often a problem to maintain the fracture in close apposition. Open reduction and internal fixation is advised (Fig. 4.112).

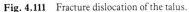

Fig. 4.111 Fracture dislocation of the talus.

Fig. 4.112 The fracture shown in Figure 4.111 after open reduction and screw fixation.

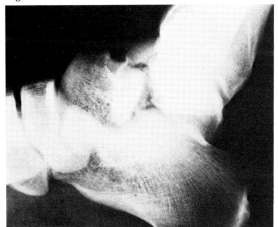

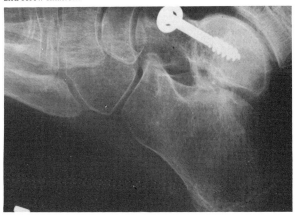

4. *Isolated fractures of the talus*
These are uncommon fractures (Fig.
4.113), mainly avulsion injuries, and
may require fixation of the
fragment, if there is considerable
separation. If there is no significant
separation, four weeks
immobilization in a short leg plaster
with a walking heel is all that is
necessary.

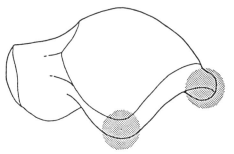

Fig. 4.113   Sites of isolated fractures of the talus.

Figure 4.114 shows a fracture of
the lateral process of the talus before
and after it has been stabilized with
wires.

Fig. 4.114   Fracture of the lateral process of the talus
before and after open reduction and K-wire fixation.

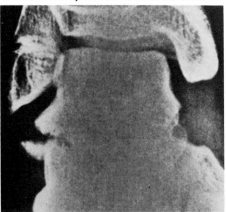

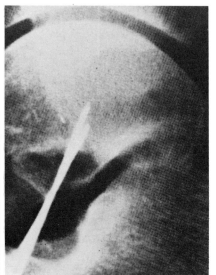

A posterior process fracture (Fig.
4.115) can be confused with a
separate ossicle, 'the os tibiale
externum'. You will need to look at
the X-rays carefully to distinguish
the two lesions − remembering that
a recent fracture has jagged edges,
and the corners are not rounded, as
with a separate ossicle . . . and, of
course with a fracture, the patient is
very tender to pressure just at that
point.

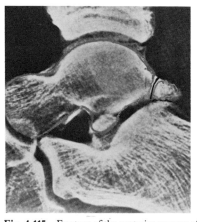

Fig. 4.115   Fracture of the posterior process of the talus.

The tarsal bones

These bones bridge from the hindfoot to the forefoot (Fig. 4.126) and as they are not very mobile bones they are not often injured.

However, injuries to each of the tarsal bones is possible with direct injury from a falling object. Twisting injuries can also cause some fractures.

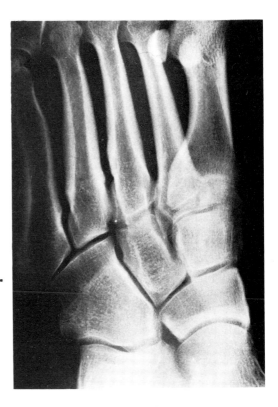

Fig. 4.126 The tarsal bones. Cub.=Cuboid; Nav.=navicular; Cun.=cuneiform.

Probably the most common of these fractures are the fractures of the cuboid and the navicular (Fig. 4.127a, 4.127b).

Fig. 4.127 Crush fracture and fracture dislocation of the navicular.

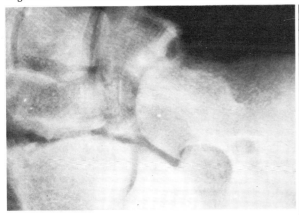
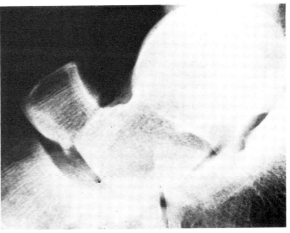

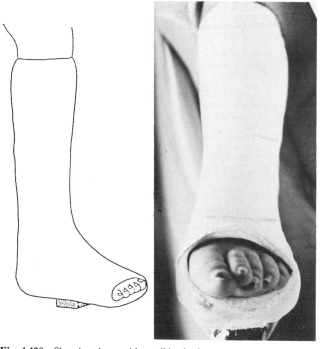

Sometimes the fracture is best seen on tomograms.

Generally, undisplaced fractures require a short leg plaster and a walking heel (Fig. 4.128a & b) for about four weeks and then limited activity for four to six weeks.

Displaced fractures of the tarsal bones and fracture dislocations require open reduction and internal fixation (Fig. 4.129a & b).

Fig. 4.128   Short leg plaster with a walking heel.

Fig. 4.129(a)   Displaced fracture of the navicular.   **(b)** Open reduction and screw fixation of (a).

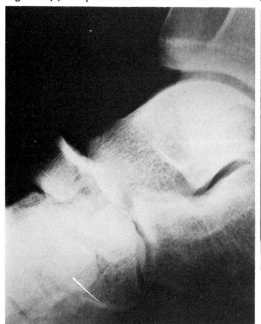

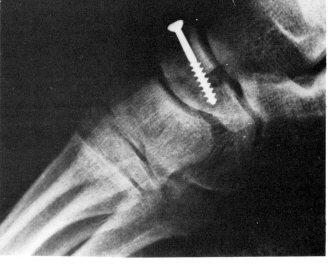

The metatarsal bones

These fractures are quite common, and many occur as a result of a heavy object falling on the foot, causing local damage to one or more of the metatarsals (Fig. 4.130).

Twisting injuries (Fig. 4.131) are responsible for the commonest fracture of the metatarsals, i.e. the fracture of the base of the fifth metatarsal. This injury occurs when the foot is twisted into inversion and contraction of the peroneus brevis muscle avulses the base of the fifth metatarsal (Fig. 4.132), sometimes with considerable displacement.

Severe twisting injuries, such as occur in a fall from a horse with the foot caught in the stirrup, are also responsible for the more serious fracture dislocation of the tarso-metatarsal joint. This is dealt with in the section of *Lisfranc's dislocation* in Chapter 5.

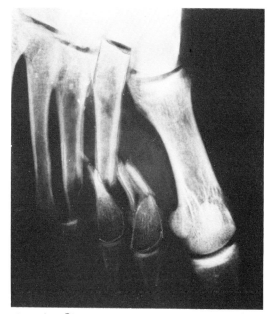

Fig. 4.130 Displaced fractures of the metatarsals caused by a direct injury.

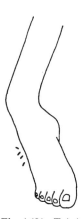

Fig. 4.131 Twisting (inversion) injury can cause a fracture of the base of the fifth metatarsal.

Fig. 4.132 Undisplaced fracture of the base of the fifth metatarsal.

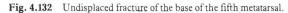

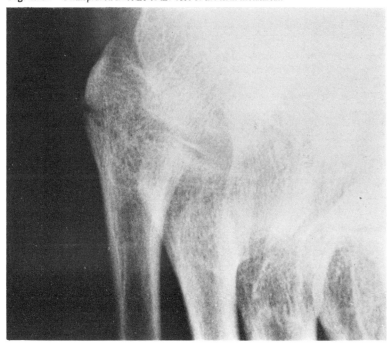

The so called 'March fracture' occurs as a stress fracture without major trauma, after prolonged and unaccustomed walking or running. It may not be picked up initially, because there is no history of trauma. Classically, it affects the second metatarsal (Fig. 4.133) and produces prolific callus. The lump of callus may be the first thing you see on X-ray (Fig. 4.134), it is diagnostic of a stress fracture.

Fig. 4.133   Diagram of March fracture, a stress fracture of the second or third metatarsal.

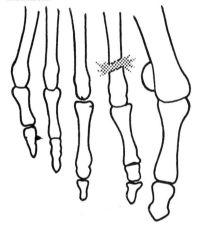

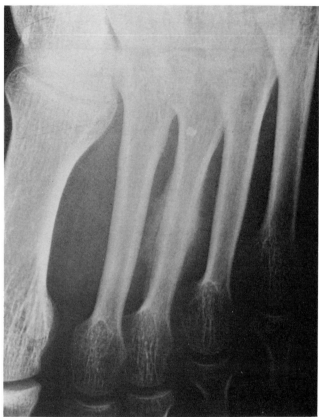

Fig. 4.134   X-ray of typical 'March' fracture.

Treatment of metatarsal fractures

These fractures are generally quite painful. When they are painful, they are best treated in a short leg plaster with a walking heel. This will be required for approximately four weeks, followed by restricted activity for a further four weeks. Apply a short leg plaster slab initially and supply crutches. Then convert this to a walking plaster after a few days.

'March' fractures and undisplaced fractures of the fifth metatarsal base

Especially with these fractures, some patients will not have much pain and discomfort after the first 24 to 48 hours. In these patients, crutches for a few days and firm support for a few weeks is sufficient treatment.

*Displaced fractures of the base of the
fifth metatarsal*

These fractures (Fig. 4.135) may
require open reduction and pinning
using K-Wires or tension band
wiring or a lag screw (Fig. 4.136).

Fractures of the fifth metatarsal
which are more distal are sometimes
slow to unite . . . (the so called Jones
fracture).

Fig. 4.135   Displaced fracture of the base
of the fifth metatarsal.

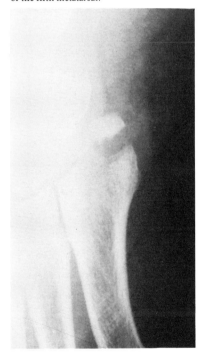

Fig. 4.136   Open reduction and screw fixation of the fracture
shown in Figure 4.135 − the screw is a little too long.

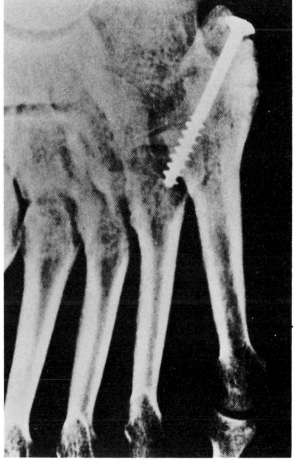

*Multiple displaced fractures of the
shafts of the metatarsals (Fig. 4.137)*

These may require percutaneous
pinning or open reduction and
pinning (Fig. 4.138) as gross
instability may be present.
Malunion of these fractures may
cause persistent pain in the forefoot.

Fig. 4.137 Multiple fractures of the metatarsals.

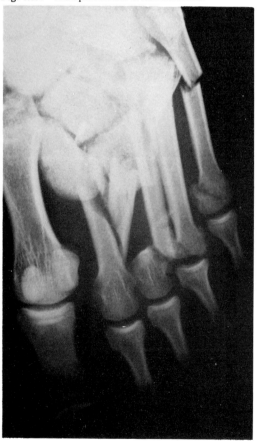

Fig. 4.138 Reduction and pin fixation of multiple fractures of the
metatarsal bones shown in Figure 4.137.

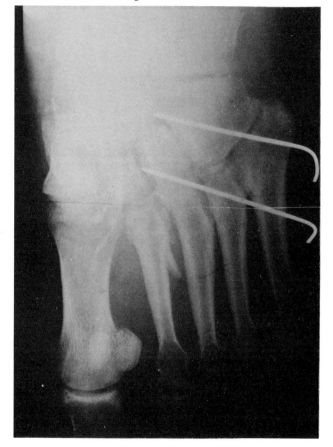

The phalanges of the toes

With the exception of the proximal phalanx of the big toe, these fractures (whilst uncomfortable) are not major problems.

The common causes of this injury are: an object falling on the foot; an accidental kick on an immovable object; or the foot being crushed in a 'run over' incident.

Management

Displaced fractures of the proximal phalanx of the big toe will require reduction – usually closed and may then require a short leg plaster. Occasionally open reduction and pinning of this fracture is required.

Most toe fractures are undisplaced (Fig. 4.139a and b) – displaced fractures can usually be reduced under local anaesthetic toe block (see Chapter 1).

Toe fractures can be treated in strapping (Fig. 4.140), with shoes that have the toes cut out and perhaps the use of crutches for a few days.

Fig 4.139   Undisplaced comminuted fracture of (a) Proximal phalanx of the big toe; (b) Distal phalanx of the big toe.

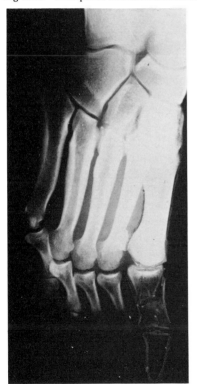

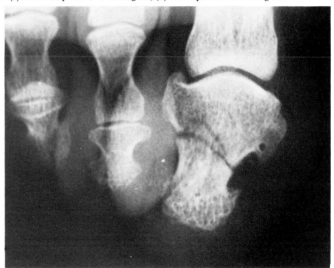

Fig. 4.140   Strapping for toe fractures.

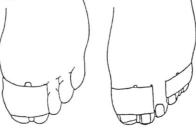
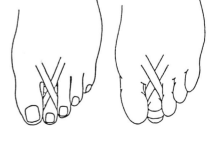

CHAPTER FIVE

Dislocations

General remarks

A dislocation of a joint usually occurs suddenly and as a result of considerable force; the exception being recurrent dislocation, where the ligamentous structures are already damaged and the joint can come out of place with minimal force.

Definitions: A Dislocation is the displacement of one or more of the bones comprising a joint. It is complete and absolute like pregnancy.

Subluxation is partial displacement or disruption of a joint.

A dislocated joint is very painful and needs to be reduced as soon as possible. Many dislocated fingers, shoulders and kneecaps are put back in place on the football field. **It does not make sense for a patient to be kept waiting for hours whilst a radiographer is summoned to tell you what your clinical assessment has already established. If you are sure that it is a dislocation and not a fracture then give it a pull**

in casualty and reduce the dislocation and save the patient hours of agony.

You will need to give the patient some intravenous pethidine and diazepam (Valium), and it is important to have the area X-rayed **after** the reduction to:

1. **Confirm the reduction;** and
2. **See that there is no associated fracture.**

Some would argue that it is unwise to reduce a dislocation before an X-ray is taken. This depends on the availability of X-ray facilities and the clinical experience and judgement of the casualty officer.

Remember that to dislocate a joint you must tear the ligaments that hold the joint in place, and these must be given time to repair. In some cases operative repair may be necessary, especially if the dislocation is a recurrent one.

Some dislocations are associated with fractures of the margins of the joint and these will often require internal fixation.

Dislocation in the upper limb

Fingers and thumb

Both the distal interphalangeal (I.P.) joint and the proximal interphalangeal joints of the fingers and the interphalangeal joint of the thumb can be dislocated easily. Many cricket and baseball players are injured in this way.

The players usually reduce the dislocations themselves (Fig. 5.1). If they do not, then a pull along the line of the finger followed by flexion of the distal portion of the digit will reduce the dislocation.

Quite a good trick is to put some Elastoplast on the digit, so that you can grip it without slipping.

It should be possible to reduce these dislocations quickly and without anaesthetic. If difficulties arise, then there is probably button-holing of the head of the phalanx through the capsule − a general anaesthetic and open reduction may be necessary.

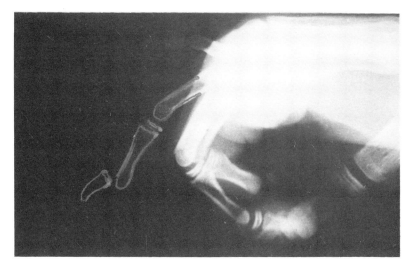

Immobilization for three weeks is necessary to allow capsular repair. Splint the finger, or thumb, on a padded aluminium splint with the finger in the semiflexed 'position of function' (Fig. 5.2).

The 'position of function' is an important concept in hand injuries. It is the relaxed position that your hand adopts when you just let it hang. N.B. The little finger is more flexed than the index finger. If the joint is stable in the 'position of function', then this is the preferred position in which to splint the fracture or dislocation.

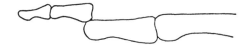

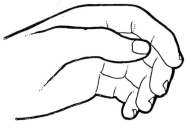

Fig. 5.2 Position of function.

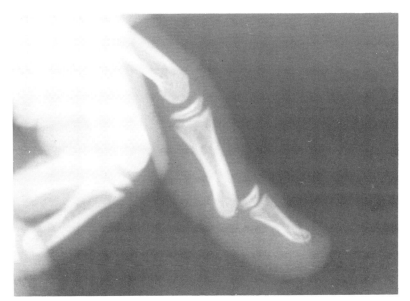

Fig. 5.1 Dislocations of the phalanges.

Metacarpo-phalangeal dislocations

Metacarpo-phalangeal dislocations
(Figs. 5.3 and 5.4) are not as
common as dislocations of the
interphalangeal joints. It is not
unusual for the joint to be difficult
to reduce due to button-holing of the
head of the metacarpal through the
capsule. **Open reduction may be
necessary.**

Closed reduction, when possible,
is obtained as described above, and
splinting on a padded aluminium
strip is necessary for three weeks.
Active exercises and physiotherapy,
in the form of wax baths and faradic
hand baths, may be helpful in
reducing the swelling and regaining
function.

BUT BEWARE!
**There are a few traps for the
unwary, even with something as
simple as a dislocated finger:**

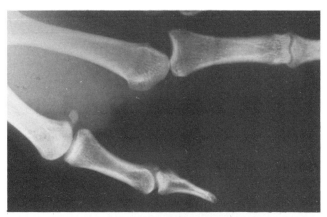

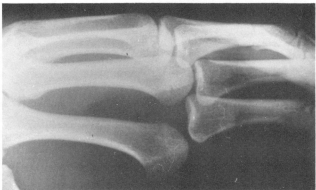

Fig. 5.3 Dislocation of the metacarpo-phalangeal (M-P) joint of the
index finger – it may be irreducible by closed means.

Fig. 5.4 Dislocation of the M-P joint of the thumb.

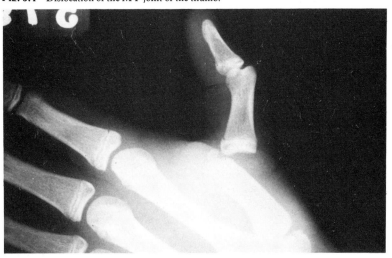

1. *The dislocation that is not a dislocation*

This is usually a young child, who is brought in with a thumb that has its tip bent over and the parents say that he doesn't move it. The thumb is not dislocated. The child has a 'trigger thumb' (Fig. 5.5) due to a lump on the flexor tendon – feel for it at the base of the thumb on the flexor surface.

The treatment for this problem is to release the mouth of the tendon sheath by operation.

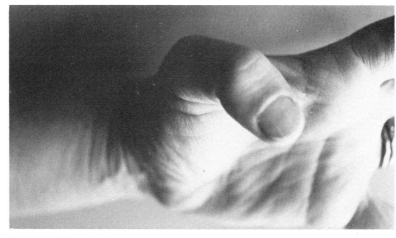

Fig. 5.5   Trigger thumb.

2. *A 'Mallet' finger (Fig. 5.6)*

This occurs when either the extensor tendon insertion is avulsed from the bone, or the piece of bone into which the tendon is inserted is avulsed.

In either case, the finger droops at the distal joint and active extension is not possible because the extensor mechanism is not intact. It will require splintage or operative repair. See the section on *Mallet fingers* in Chapter 6.

Fig. 5.6   Mallet finger.

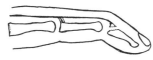
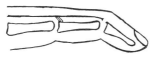

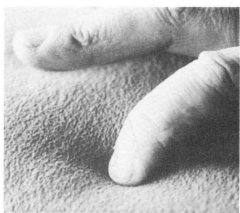

3. *Finally beware of the boutonnière deformity (Fig. 5.7)* or button-holing of the proximal I.P. joint to the uninitiated.

This may also look like a dislocation. In fact, it is a flexion deformity of the proximal I.P. joint due to damage to the extensor mechanism – namely, the central slip of the extensor tendon as it inserts into the base of the middle phalanx.

Fig. 5.7   Boutonnière deformity.

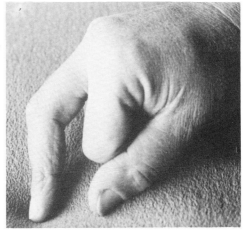

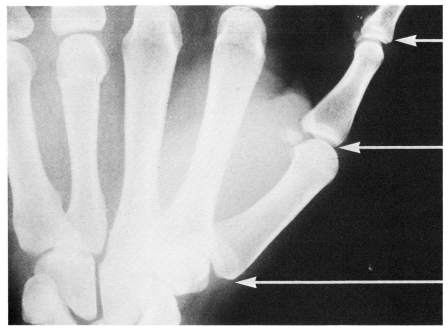

Fig. 5.8   The joints of the thumb.

Carpo-metacarpal joints

These are rare, with the exception of the carpo-metacarpal joint of the thumb; in which case, it is usually combined with a fracture of the base of the metacarpal and is called a **Bennett's fracture**. It is really a fracture dislocation − see the section on fracture of the *Metacarpals* in Chapter 2.

A lot of people when looking at X-rays casually, mistake the carpo-metacarpal joint of the thumb for the meta-carpophalangeal joint. Remember there is only ONE interphalangeal joint in the thumb (Fig. 5.8).

Dislocations at the carpo-metacarpal joint of the fingers or thumb usually require regional or general anaesthesia for reduction. **Subluxations** of these joints can be pushed back with gentle pressure without anaesthesia.

Complete dislocations of the carpo-metacarpal joints (Fig. 5.9) are usually unstable and require percutaneous pinning.

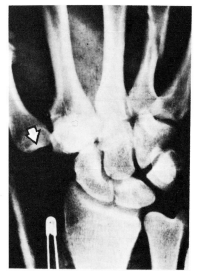

Fig. 5.9   Dislocation of the carpo-metacarpal joint of the thumb.

The carpus – wrist

It is very rare for the carpus as a whole to dislocate, but it can happen and is easy to detect on X-rays – reduce under anaesthesia and retain in plaster.

Dislocations of the lunate

A much more common, interesting and challenging dislocation is that of the lunate.

It is a lesion that is commonly missed on the X-ray; although it is obvious, *if* you look at the lateral view of the wrist and always check that the carpal bones are in one horizontal plane and not two.

Figure 5.10 shows the normal position of the carpus, in one layer, whereas Figures 5.11 and 5.12 have two layers. The lunate is dislocated in Figure 5.11, but what is the situation in Figure 5.12?

Please recheck Figures 5.10, 5.11 and 5.12 and be sure you understand this point. When you look at an X-ray of the wrist this is one of the first things you must **always check.**

Sometimes these patients will complain of numbness and tingling in the distribution of the median nerve and this should alert you to doubly check the position of the lunate; because when it dislocates, it always dislocates anteriorly and therefore presses the median nerve hard up against the anterior wall of the carpal tunnel.

If you fail to pick up the dislocation initially, the patient will complain of a lot of pain and be distressed by the severity of it.

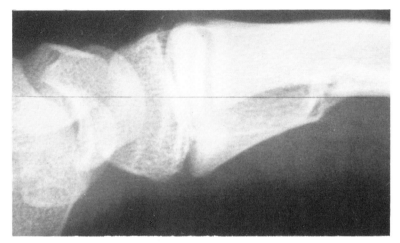

Fig. 5.10   Is the lunate or the carpus dislocated? No.

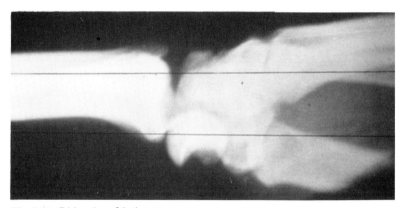

Fig. 5.11   Dislocation of the lunate.

Fig. 5.12   Is the lunate dislocated?
No, but the rest of the carpal bones and half the scaphoid are. *See* p. 29.

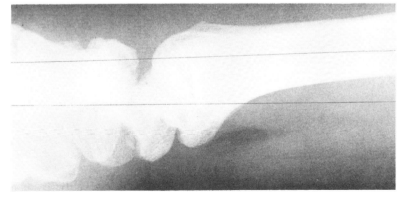

Median nerve symptoms, even if not present initially will occur within 24-48 hours and there will be **a great deal of swelling in the hand.**

N.B. You may well have missed a dislocated lunate if:

1. The patient has an abnormal amount of post injury pain.

2. The patient has pain, tingling and numbness in the median nerve distribution area.

3. The patient has more swelling than one would expect.

X-rays of a perilunate dislocation, in which the lunate is in place and the rest of the carpus is dislocated, are shown in Figure 2.42 of Chapter 2.

The elbow – children and adults

Elbow dislocations (Figs. 5.13 and 5.14) are not a difficult problem. Reduction of the dislocation, as soon as anaesthesia can be arranged, is all that is required.

Technique

When the patient is relaxed under anaesthesia, traction is applied to the hand with the forearm supinated. Maintain the traction and slowly flex the elbow. The joint should reduce and be stable in flexion.

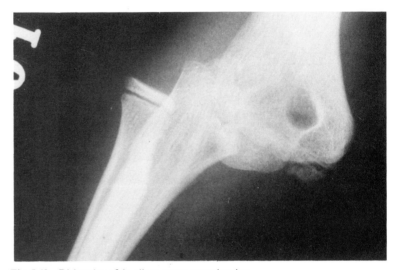

Fig. 5.13   Dislocation of the elbow, antero-posterior view.

Fig. 5.14   Dislocation of the elbow, lateral view.

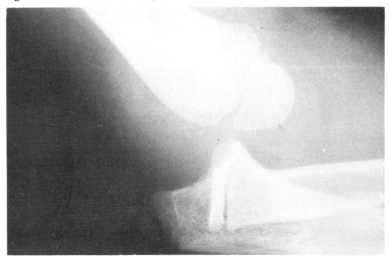

N.B. If the elbow reduces but you are unable to flex it fully, then there is a bone fragment jamming in the joint. In children, this will often be the epiphysis of the medial epicondyle (see Fig. 2.92). In adults, it can be a piece of the head of the radius or a piece of the capitellum.

In this case, open surgery will be necessary to move the bony fragment caught in the joint. Prior to operation, immobilize the elbow in a long arm plaster slab.

After reduction, immobilize the arm in an inside collar and cuff for three weeks and then **active movements** can be started. **Passive movements and forced movements and carrying heavy weights are not permitted. They will increase stiffness.**

In an adult, it is not unusual for there to be 10-15 degrees loss of flexion and extension, and about one third loss of pronation and supination. **This loss may be permanent.**

Shoulder joint

This is the most common joint dislocation (Fig. 5.15)

The patient will usually tell you what is wrong as they come into the room hanging onto the arm at the wrist and holding the limb close to the body to stop movement.

You will see at a glance that the patient has lost the roundness of the shoulder (Figs. 5.16 and 5.17). This is due to the head of the humerus not being in place. Instead there is a flatness and, on palpation, a prominence of the acromion and coracoid processes. All movements will be resisted as they are painful.

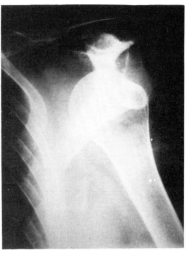

Fig. 5.15 Dislocation of the shoulder.

Fig. 5.16 The clinical picture of a shoulder dislocation − note the loss of contour of the shoulder.

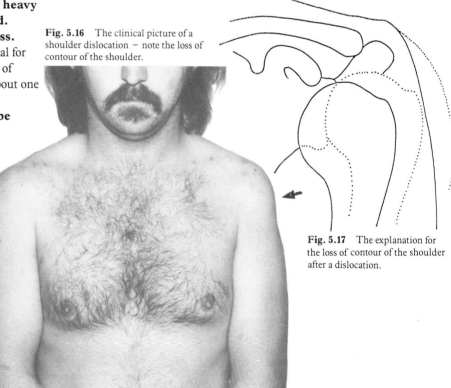

Fig. 5.17 The explanation for the loss of contour of the shoulder after a dislocation.

Treatment

What you do next depends on being sure of your diagnosis. If you are confident, and especially if it is a recurrent dislocation in a person of slight build, then you should reduce the dislocation forthwith. No delay, because delay here means pain for the patient.

Give the patient a suitable dose of pethedine and diazepam (Valium) intravenously.

Reduce the dislocation by: traction in slight abduction (Fig. 5.18), with countertraction in the axilla from your assistant; external rotation (Fig. 5.19); and then adduction (Fig. 5.20) and internal rotation (Fig. 5.21). Usually before the manoeuvres are complete, the shoulder gently pops in. Finally, support the arm with an inside collar and cuff.

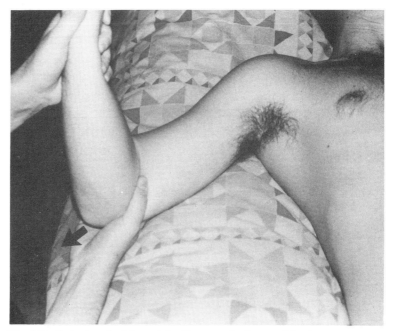

Fig. 5.18   Reduction of a dislocated shoulder − traction in some abduction.

Fig. 5.19   External rotation whilst still keeping up the traction.

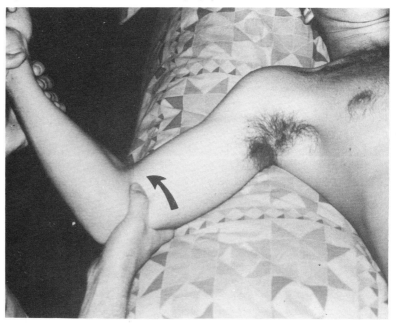

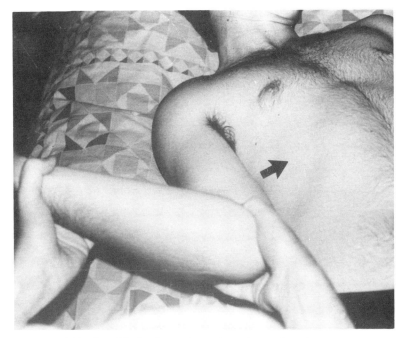

Fig. 5.20 Adduction whilst keeping up the traction and external rotation.

Fig. 5.21 Internal rotation sweeping the hand across the chest.

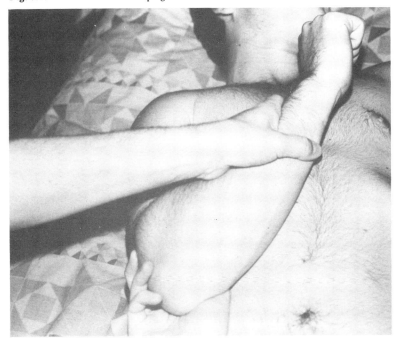

In most cases reduction is really easy, provided that traction is maintained for a minute or two.

You may have difficulty in reducing the shoulder in very muscular people – especially if it is their first dislocation.

If you are unable to reduce the dislocation by this method, sometimes you can reduce the shoulder by hanging the unsupported arm over the side of a bed with the patient holding a 4kg weight in the hand (Fig. 5.22) while they are still under the influence of the analgesics. In this position their muscles will relax and the shoulder will reduce.

If both these methods are unsuccessful, then you are out of luck and the patient will need a general anaesthetic and reduction as above.

You should X-ray the patient to confirm the reduction (Fig. 5.23).

N.B. There can be an associated fracture of the greater tuberosity.

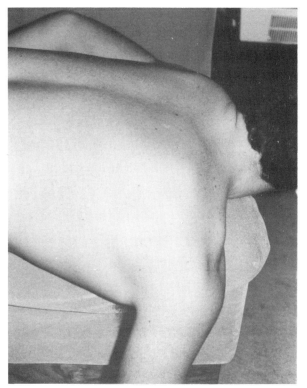

Fig. 5.22   Reduction by hanging the arm over the edge of a table with a weight in the hand.

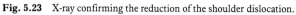

Fig. 5.23   X-ray confirming the reduction of the shoulder dislocation.

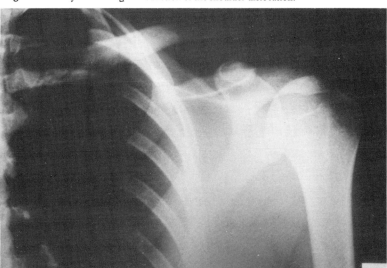

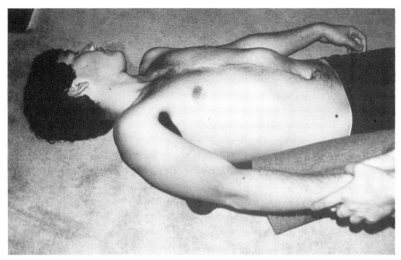

Fig. 5.24 The Hippocratic method of reduction of a dislocated shoulder.

The 'Hippocratic method' of reduction (Fig. 5.24) is not recommended as it can damage the nerve supply to the deltoid.

Please check the function of the axillary (circumflex) nerve which supplies the motor power for the deltoid muscle – ask the patient to gently abduct the shoulder.

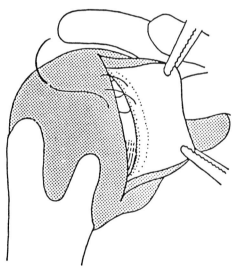

Fig. 5.25 The principle of the Putti-Platt operation – double-breasting the capsule.

Problems with dislocated shoulders

1. Recurrent dislocation
A dislocation is technically recurrent when it has occurred for the second time. However, most surgeons would be reluctant to operate on a patient after only two dislocations, especially if they have both occurred with a reasonable amount of force.

An operation is necessary if the shoulder has come out more than twice and especially if it has dislocated with minimal force. **In this case, you must reduce the dislocation and book the patient in to see an orthopaedic surgeon, who will arrange an operation to repair the capsule.**

The most widely used surgical technique was described by two surgeons at the same time and is known by both their names, Vittoro Putti and Sir Harry Platt, hence the Putti-Platt operation (Fig. 5.25).

2. *Missed dislocation*

Occasionally a dislocation is overlooked, or a patient fails to come for attention, and a dislocation is left unreduced for several weeks. Surprisingly, some of these can be reduced by closed means provided prolonged traction and countertraction is used.

In little old ladies take care not to fracture the shaft of the humerus. Remember all long bones are more vulnerable when subjected to twisting (torsional) forces.

Open reduction can be carried out, and care is needed to avoid damage to the nerves and vessels of the axilla.

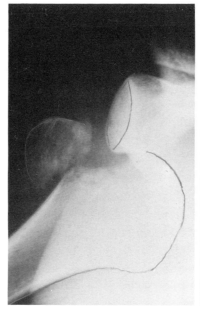
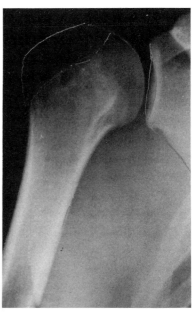

Fig. 5.26   A fracture dislocation of the shoulder (a) before and (b) after reduction.

3. *Dislocations with fractures*

The fracture shown in Fig. 5.26a will hopefully reduce into place (as shown in Fig. 5.26b) when the dislocation is reduced. The most common associated fracture is that of the greater tuberosity, and usually it does slip into place. However, if there is still displacement (Fig. 5.27a) after reduction of the dislocation, **then open reduction and internal fixation of the fracture is necessary (Fig. 5.27b).**

Fig. 5.27(a)   A fracture dislocation. **(b)** Methods of internal fixation.

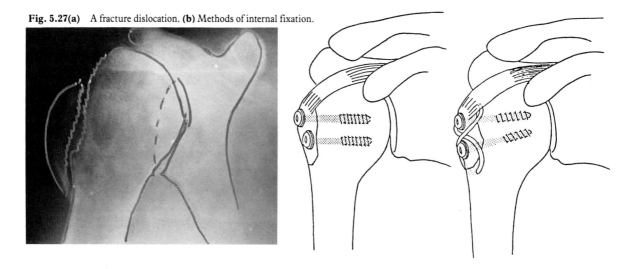

4. *Dislocations with nerve damage*
While it is possible to damage the brachial plexus in the same injury that dislocates the shoulder, this is rare. Usually, the injury that damages a brachial plexus is a violent one and it more often causes a fracture of the humerus than a dislocation of the shoulder. **Always test for major nerve damage.**

Quick tests:
  a. Thumbs up − radial nerve (Fig. 5.28)
  b. Fingers spread out − ulnar nerve (Fig. 5.29)
  c. Thumb and little finger opposed − median nerve (Fig. 5.30).

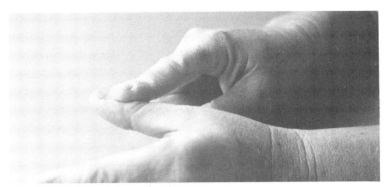

Fig. 5.28 Testing radial nerve function.

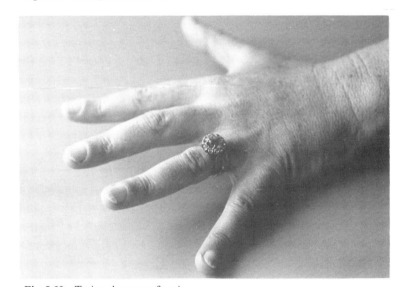

Fig. 5.29 Testing ulnar nerve function.

Fig. 5.30 Testing median nerve function.

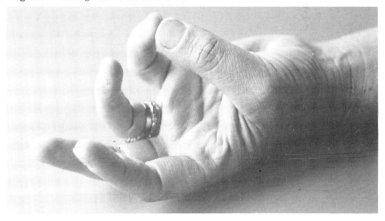

Sensory function should be tested and the patterns of sensory loss of the radial, ulnar and median nerve can be charted as shown in Fig. 5.31.

In a dislocation of the shoulder, the axillary (circumflex) nerve is most frequently damaged. Test this nerve by testing abduction of the shoulder — is the deltoid muscle working?

The axillary (circumflex) nerve is in immediate inferior relation to the shoulder joint and can be stretched and even avulsed in a dislocation. Usually, it is only stretched and has neuropraxia (goes on strike) for a few weeks.

An important prognostic sign is to see if sensation is absent over the area of the insertion of the deltoid (Fig. 5.32):

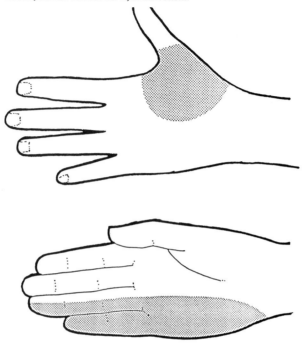

Fig. 5.31 Testing for loss of sensation: the radial nerve, at the top: the ulnar nerve, in the middle; and the median nerve, at the bottom.

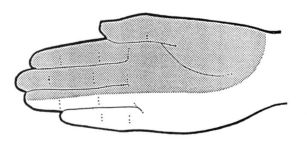

Fig. 5.32 Patch of anaesthesia in axillary nerve damage.

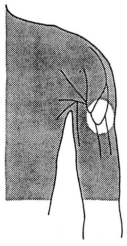

1. **If sensation is present, motor power will return to the deltoid in about three weeks;**
2. **If there is an area of anaesthesia present, it will be a valuable guide to recovery — if it stays, then there will be no recovery, but if it disappears, recovery is three weeks away.**

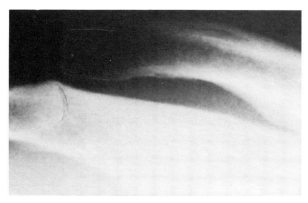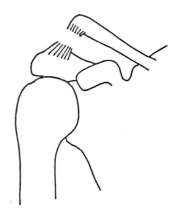

Fig. 5.33 Complete dislocation of the acromio-clavicular joint.

Acromio-clavicular dislocations

Injuries to this joint are common, but dislocations of the joint are not as common (Fig. 5.33) as subluxations (Fig. 5.34).

The injury is caused by a fall on the point of the shoulder, and comes in three grades:
  'sprung' joint;
  'subluxed' joint; and
  'dislocated' joint.

1. *The sprung joint* is a common injury and is characterized by pain and swelling over the acromioclavicular and a normal X-ray. Treatment is limited to a two week rest from football and other active sports and a sling until the soreness goes.

2. *Subluxation of the acromio-clavicular joint* is also common and also has pain and swelling over the joint. On X-ray under stress, i.e.

carrying a weight, the outer end of the clavicle rides up. **Treatment is three weeks in a sling (Fig. 5.35) – not a collar and cuff, as the elbow needs to be supported.**

Fig. 5.34 Subluxation of the acromio-clavicular (A-C) joint.

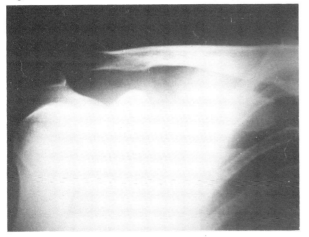

Fig. 5.35 The sling must support tightly under the elbow.

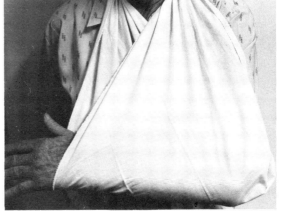

Another way to support the elbow and hold the subluxation in place is with non-elastic strapping and a pad over the acromio-clavicular joint and around under the elbow (Fig. 5.36).

3. *Dislocation of the acromio-clavicular joint (Fig. 5.33)* is often due to a heavy fall on the point of the shoulder.

Treatment of this injury calls for internal fixation of the joint with wires (Fig. 5.37) or with a coraco-clavicular screw and perhaps repair or replacement of the ligaments.

There is one school of thought, that suggests that the patient be treated in a sling for three weeks, and then has active use of the arm and assessment to see if the patient will accept the cosmetic and functional disability.

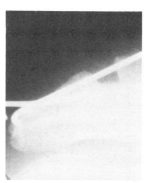

Fig. 5.37 Strong K-wires for fixation of acromio-clavicular joint.

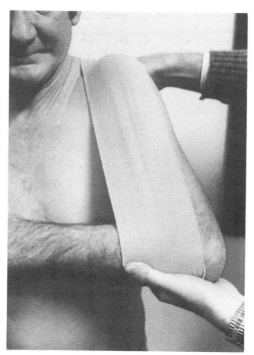

Fig. 5.36 Non-stretch strapping under the elbow and over the A-C joint – pad both these areas.

Sterno-clavicular joint

This joint is well protected by its position and strong ligamentous attachments.

It is possible to have four types of injury to this joint:

1. *A fracture* of the inner end of the clavicle involving the joint. For treatment details see the sections on *Fractures of the Clavicle* and *Fractures of the Sternum* in Chapter 3.

2. *A 'sprain' of the joint* – a partial rupture of the anterior ligaments. Clinically the joint is in place, but there is pain on movement and some swelling of the area with localized tenderness to pressure over the joint. Treatment is simply a sling and limited activity for ten days.

3. *Anterior dislocation* in which the medial end of the clavicle is levered out of its socket by a heavy blow to the anterior aspect of the shoulder whilst the arm is in the abducted position. The diagnosis is usually obvious, as there is a large lump at the site of the joint and this is very tender. Gentle pressure on the clavicle will allow reduction, and holding the arm in a sling *in front of the body* will keep the dislocation reduced. A figure of eight bandage (see Fig. 3.6 in Ch. 3) is advocated by some, but will tend to allow the joint to redislocate.

Open reduction is indicated only in irreducible and chronic dislocations.

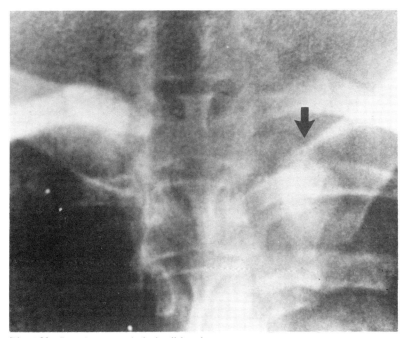

Fig. 5.38 Posterior sterno-clavicular dislocation.

4. *Posterior dislocations* (Fig. 5.38) are fortunately rare, as the inner end of the clavicle can press on the great vessels and/or the trachea. The injury occurs as a result of a heavy and direct blow on the anterior aspect of the inner end of the clavicle, which then goes retrosternally. The injury can result in death on the football field.

Recognition of the injury is not difficult as the patient is distressed and in severe pain over the sternum. **If there is dyspnoea then reduction is urgent as there is pressure on the trachea.** The clavicle is shortened as it disappears behind the sternum.

Reduction is not difficult, as a rule, provided the lesion is not left for more than 24 hours – after this it becomes difficult and open reduction and fixation may be necessary.

Closed reduction is achieved by pulling both shoulders back – **any drop in blood pressure may indicate some damage in the chest, therefore be prepared and have a trolley with all the appropriate resuscitation equipment on hand.**

The joint should be immobilized in a figure of eight bandage (see Fig. 3.6 in Ch. 3) for three weeks.

Dislocations of the lower limb

The hip joint

Your role in the casualty department, as far as this injury is concerned, is to recognize this injury and to arrange prompt reduction of the dislocated hip by a competent registrar or an orthopaedic surgeon.

Reduction is not difficult as a rule, but it does require quite a lot of strength and some skill. The real problem for the casualty officer who attempts the reduction is what to do if the hip does not go back.

What is the clinical and X-ray picture? There are three anatomical types of dislocation − posterior dislocation occurs at more than twice the frequency of the other types combined.

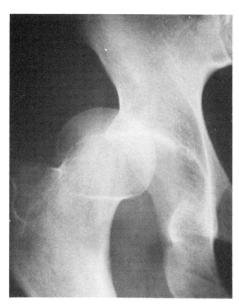

Fig. 5.39 Posterior dislocation of the hip.

Fig. 5.40 The clinical picture of a posterior dislocation of the hip.

1. Posterior dislocation (Figs. 5.39 and 5.40)

In posterior dislocations of the hip there is shortening of the leg, adduction of the thigh and internal rotation of the leg (Fig. 5.39) − all due to the position of the head of the femur. **The picture is different if there is a fracture of the femoral shaft as well as a dislocated hip (Fig. 1.4), for then the adduction of the leg, and the rotation are corrected at the fracture site.** That is why you must always be able to see the hip joint on the X-rays of a fracture of the shaft of the femur. See *Looking at X-rays* in Chapter 1.

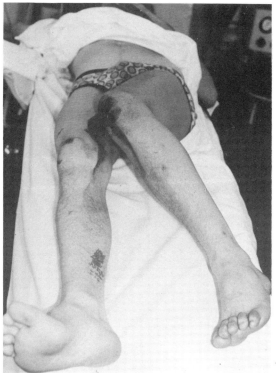

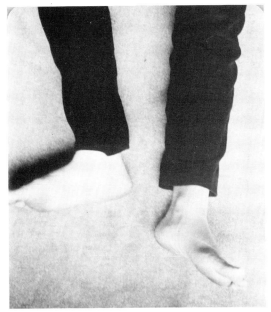

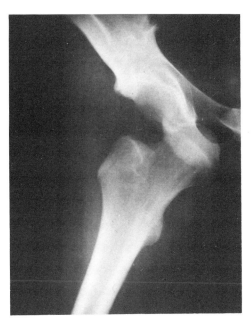

Fig. 5.41 The clinical picture of an anterior dislocation of the hip – note that the knee is flexed, hence the leg looks shorter.

Fig. 5.42 X-ray of an anterior dislocation of the hip.

2. Anterior dislocation (Figs. 5.41 and 5.42)

In this type of dislocation of the hip, the leg is abducted (up to ninety degrees) but not shortened – except that the knee is usually partly flexed (Fig. 5.41).

3. Central dislocation

This is a really severe fracture of the pelvis with displacement of the head of the femur through the shattered acetabular floor (Fig. 5.43).

This injury is often only one of many suffered by the patient – they are almost always car accident victims and the force necessary to cause this type of fracture usually breaks limbs and causes head and abdominal injuries.

Fig. 5.43 Central dislocation of the hip.

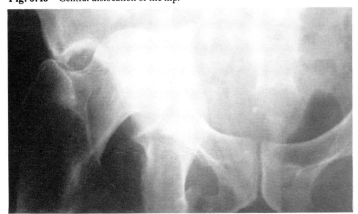

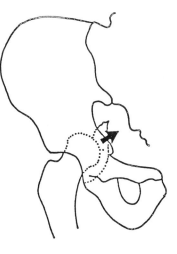

If this patient is shocked then suspect visceral injury – all patients who have fractures of the pelvis must be checked to see if there has been a bladder injury.

They must be asked to void. If they can't, then they should be catheterised and the urine must be checked for blood. If there is any doubt, a cystogram is done without delay.

This patient will be admitted to hospital and definitive treatment of the pelvic injury and the central dislocation will depend on a number of factors – such as the associated injuries and the general condition of the patient.

Generally, treatment consists of reduction of the dislocation by traction and the maintenance of the traction until the floor of the acetabulum has healed.

Lateral traction, through a Green screw inserted in the neck of the femur (Fig. 5.44), is more effective than traction through the femoral shaft or the tibia.

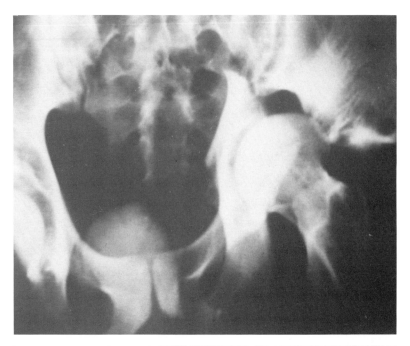

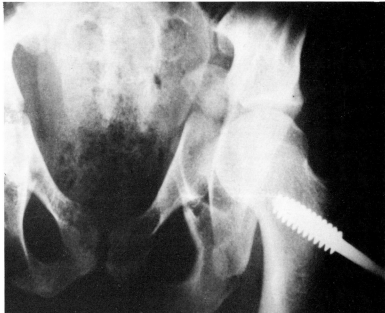

Fig. 5.44   Central dislocation of the hip before and after lateral traction through a Green screw.

Reduction of a dislocated hip

The mechanics of reducing a
dislocated hip by several methods is
shown below:

1. *Traction with the hip and knee
flexed, and leg leverage (Fig. 5.45)*
Note that in this method the patient
is anaesthetised and relaxed and is
on a canvas on the floor to allow
better leverage. The surgeon's foot is
placed in the patient's groin, to
allow counter traction.

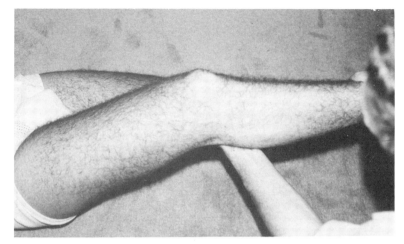

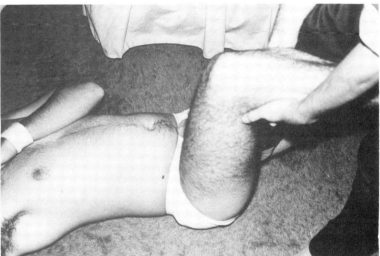

Fig. 5.45   Reduction of a dislocated hip − patient on the floor, knee flexed to 90 degrees,
foot in the groin for counter-traction.

2. *The 'Allis' method (Fig. 5.46)*
In the 'Allis' method, the patient is
on a trolley under a relaxant general
anaesthetic. The hip is reduced by
gentle levering over the surgeon's
shoulder, or using a figure-four arm
lock.

You will need to test whether the
reduction is successful – the limb
should now be the same length and
appearance as the other limb, and
should move freely at the hip joint.

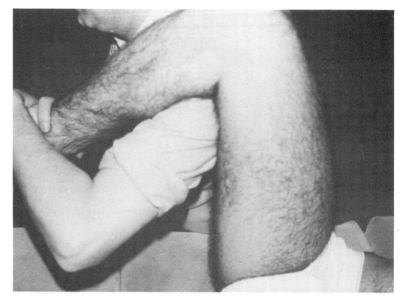

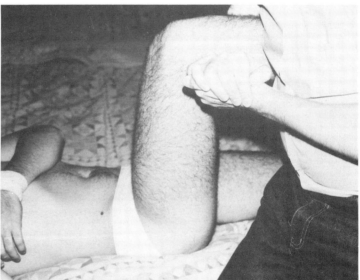

Fig. 5.46   The Allis method of reduction of a dislocated hip.

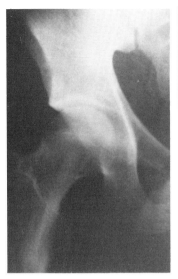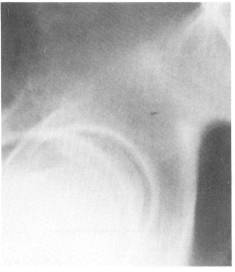

Fig. 5.47 Antero-posterior and lateral views of the hip to confirm reduction.

Look at the X-rays carefully.
Have you reduced the hip
successfully? If you have then you
should be able to see the lesser
trochanter on the antero-posterior
X-ray film. If it is still dislocated,
then the leg will be internally
rotated and the lesser trochanter will
not be visible. Make sure that you
have a lateral film of the hip joint
confirming reduction (Fig. 5.47).

Problems with dislocated hips

Why can't you reduce all dislocated
hips by the above methods?
  1. There may be a fracture of the
acetabular margin (Fig. 5.48) which
may reduce first and jam in the
joint; or if the piece is large, then
you may be able to reduce the hip
but it will remain unstable as there
is insufficient support in the
postero-superior wall. In either case
open reduction is required.

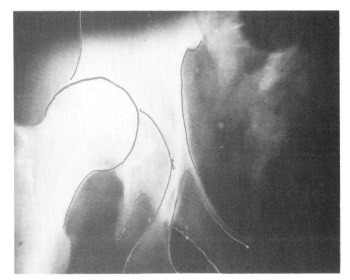

Fig. 5.48 Dislocated hip with a fractured acetabular margin.

2. Sometimes there is a fracture of the head of the femur and a small piece prevents relocation of the head (Fig. 5.49) – it will need to be removed or re-attached. Admit the patient and order blood for all these open procedures, because they are major surgical operations.

3. Occasionally, the head of the femur buttonholes through a small tear in the capsule and cannot withdraw through the same hole during closed reduction. Open reduction is therefore necessary.

In about ten per cent of cases of dislocation of the hip there is nerve damage, usually to the sciatic nerve. **Test for sciatic nerve function by testing sensation (Fig. 5.50) and power below the knee (Fig. 5.51).**

Recovery time can be slow (three to thirty months) and not all cases recover.

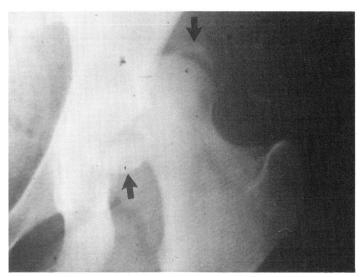

Fig. 5.49 Dislocated hip with a fracture of the head of the femur.

Fig. 5.51 Testing for power in dorsi and plantar flexion.

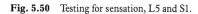

Fig. 5.50 Testing for sensation, L5 and S1.

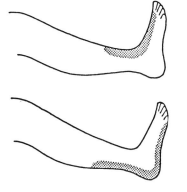

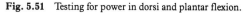

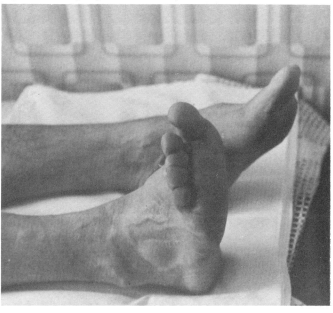

The patella

Patella dislocations are quite common and usually occur as a result of a sporting incident. The victim has the knee partially flexed and a sudden contraction of the quadriceps combined with a twisting motion dislocates the kneecap. The patella then balances unsteadily on the lateral supracondylar ridge, only to flip back into place as the knee is straightened – or it flips around to the lateral side of the femur, as shown in Figure 5.52.

Do not confuse this with the much more serious dislocated knee joint (Fig. 5.53), which occurs as a result of major trauma and in which the tibia is dislocated on the femur.

In this case, there is obvious displacement of the patella laterally with distortion of the outline of the knee joint. Since this lesion is very painful, reduction should not be delayed to obtain X-ray confirmation of what is clinically obvious.

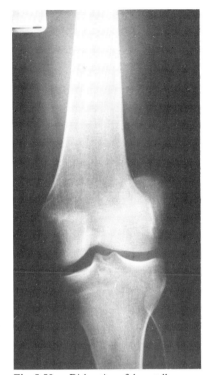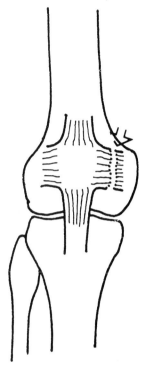

Fig. 5.52a Dislocation of the patella.
b Rupture of the vastus medialis insertion, which must accompany a lateral dislocation.

Fig. 5.53 Dislocation of the knee joint.

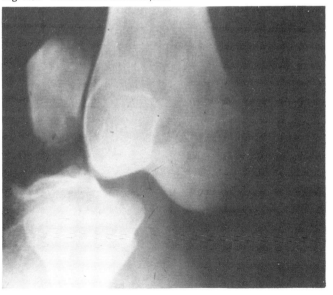

Reduction

Usually, this is easily carried out under some intravenous analgesia (pethedine and diazepam). Gently straighten the knee whilst pushing the patella medially with your thumb on its lateral border.

Immobilize the knee in a long leg plaster cylinder after X-raying the knee to confirm the reduction and to see that there is no associated fracture of the patella. Plaster immobilization should be maintained for four weeks to allow the capsule to repair.

Recurrent dislocation of the patella

About 40 per cent of dislocations of the patella are recurrent and many of these patients will require a repair operation, if they are to play sport again. For this reason, some surgeons advocate repair of the torn structures (Fig. 5.52b).

This is especially advised in serious athletes, and those with abnormally placed patellae.

The knee

This is a rare dislocation (Fig. 5.53) and can be a terrifying injury. Almost all cases that have been reported have been the result of motor vehicle accidents — usually a short pedestrian hit by a car with a high bumper bar.

Why so terrifying? Because one third of the cases have **arterial and venous damage.**

What you do **now**, may well determine the fate of this leg. If there is vascular damage, the foot will show obvious signs — being cold and pale, or blue and engorged.

Pull on the leg and reduce the dislocation. Has the circulation returned to normal? If it has not returned to normal, then arrange an arteriogram immediately (Fig. 5.54) as vascular damage has occurred and repair is essential and urgent.

In most series, about one quarter of the total number of patients with a dislocated knee end up with an amputation.

Delay in reduction and vascular repair increases the risk of amputation.

If the knee is dislocated medially or laterally, then ligamentous repair is often advised. However, if the knee is dislocated anteriorly or posteriorly, reduction and maintenance of the leg in a split plaster cast is all that is necessary.

Foot drop commonly occurs, due to damage to the lateral popliteal nerve which is stretched and often avulsed.

Fig. 5.54   A normal and an abnormal arteriogram.

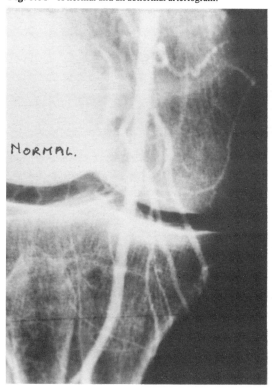
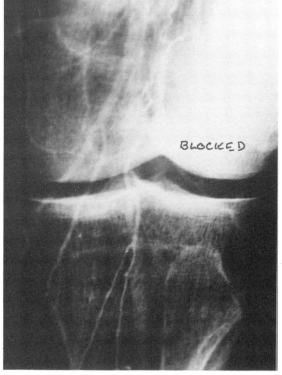

The ankle

Whilst it is not impossible to dislocate the ankle without having a fracture of the medial or lateral malleolus, it is difficult and hence the lesion is very rare (Fig. 5.55).

Check the circulation – it is often compromised and reduction is then urgent, i.e. immediately in the casualty department.

Reduction is necessary under a general anaesthetic. **Try and open up the space for the talus and then rotate the foot into alignment while maintaining strong traction.** Open reduction may be needed if the tendons on the medial or lateral sides become caught around the talus.

Fracture dislocation of the ankle

This is a common injury – see full details under *Ankle fractures* in Chapter 4.

Fig. 5.55 Dislocation of the ankle.

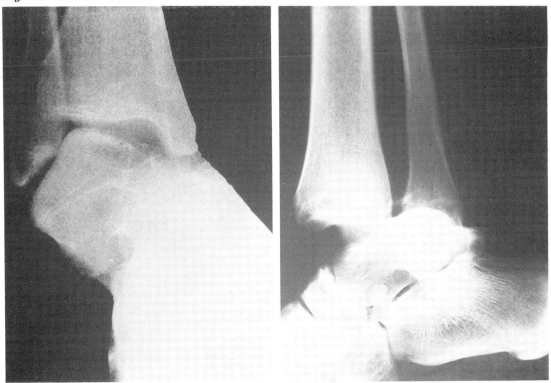

Dislocations of the subtaloid joint

Once again a rare injury (Fig. 5.56) and **almost always a compound injury.** If it is not compound, then the skin is often so tightly stretched that the area becomes devitalised very quickly – reduction is therefore a matter of urgency to save the skin.

Reduction can be difficult – one needs to assess the deformity on the X-rays and work out which way the talus and leg are lying in relation to the os calcis and foot. **Open up the subtalar joint with a levering action of both hands and then rotate the foot and heel back into line.** Often there is a lot of grinding and crunching and things pop back into place. Confirm the reduction on X-ray, apply a well padded backslab, and keep the patient in hospital for essential checks on the circulation in the foot, during the next twelve hours.

For fracture dislocations see the section on *The talus* in Chapter 4.

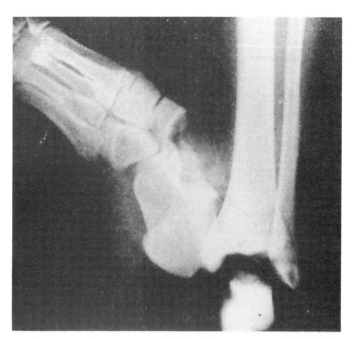
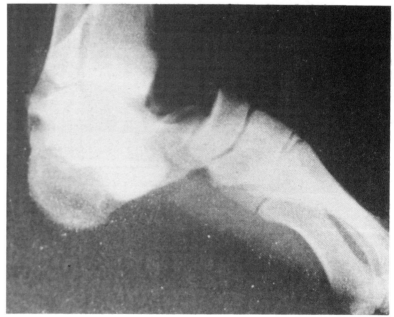

Fig. 5.56   Total dislocation of the talus – ankle and subtalar joint are dislocated.

The tarsal bones

These are the most tightly wedged in bones in the body − surely they can't be prized out of place?

Yes, they can. Figure 5.57 shows a dislocated talo-navicular joint and a dislocated navicular. Open reduction is necessary, and your primary concern will be to arrange early reduction, to preserve **skin and circulation.**

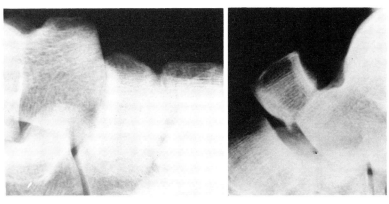

Fig. 5.57   Dislocation of the talo-navicular joint, and a dislocated navicular bone.

Tarso-metatarsal joint − Lisfranc's fracture dislocation

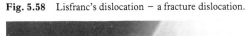

Fig. 5.58   Lisfranc's dislocation − a fracture dislocation.

Lisfranc described this injury in 1840, in cavalrymen injured on the field of battle. The dislocation (Fig. 5.58) occurred when the soldier was thrown from his horse with the foot still caught in the stirrup. Nowadays, it occurs in motor vehicle accidents, falls from a ladder, and even just tripping and catching the toes. A crushing injury can also cause this dislocation.

The circulation in the forefoot may be obstructed by direct pressure on the vessels with the metatarsals dislocated. If the toes are blue and cold, then pull on the forefoot and reduce the dislocation as best you can **as quickly as possible.** Formal reduction can then be done at a later time, as the danger to the foot has passed once the circulation has been restored.

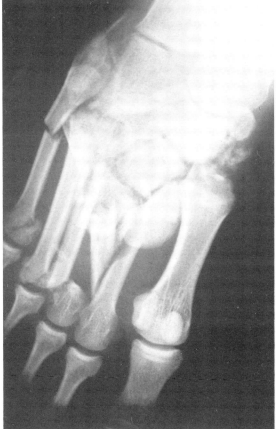

Reduction is not difficult and needs traction on the toes and direct pressure over the dislocated bones. If the reduction is unstable then percutaneous pinning with strong K-wires will be necessary. A well padded backslab, elevation of the leg and observation of the circulation in the toes (with the patient in hospital) is essential.

Problems with Lisfranc's dislocation

1. *Circulation problems* – see above.

2. *Associated fracture*
There are commonly fractures of one or more of the bases of the metatarsals and often associated fractures of the metatarsal shafts or necks, especially if there has been a crushing injury. These fractures complicate the management, especially fractures of the bases of the metatarsals as they create instability.

The dislocation is usually unstable if the first metatarsal is dislocated or fractured, and is always unstable if the second metatarsal is fractured (Fig. 5.59). Unstable fracture dislocations require reduction – closed, if possible, or open with pinning (Fig. 5.60).

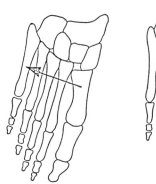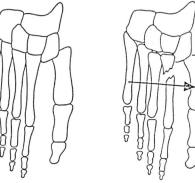

Fig. 5.59   Examples of Lisfranc's dislocations.

Fig. 5.60   Lisfranc's fracture dislocation before and after open reduction using K-wires.

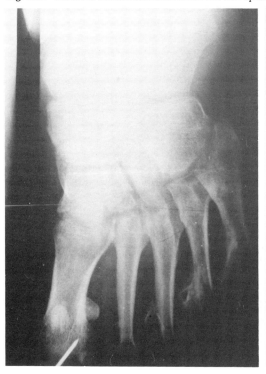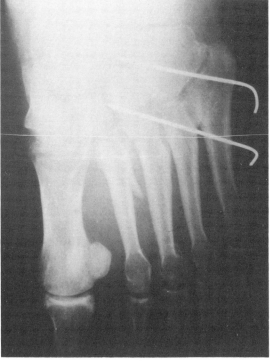

Metatarso-phalangeal joints

These joints can be dislocated by a heavy fall, and this same injury frequently causes a fracture of the neck of the metatarsal.

The dislocation is usually dorsal and reduction is by traction and flexion of the phalanx − unstable dislocations need to be pinned for three weeks.

Interphalangeal joints

Dislocations of the phalanges are common (Fig. 5.61) − usually from tripping or a misdirected kick whilst in bare feet.

Reduction is usually by traction and flexion of the toe. The toe can then be strapped to the adjacent digit for three weeks (Fig. 5.62).

Again a joint that is unstable will require a Kirschner wire across the joint for three weeks (Fig. 5.62).

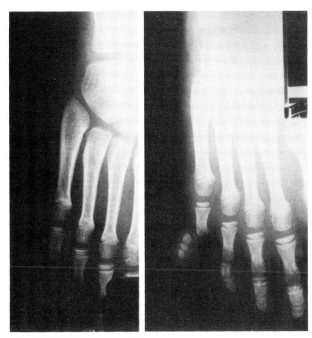

Fig. 5.61   Dislocation of a little toe.

Fig. 5.62   Strapping if the dislocation is stable or K-wire fixation if unstable.

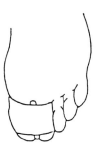 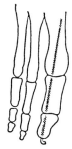

CHAPTER SIX

Tendon injuries

Rupture of the Achilles' tendon

Rupture of the Achilles' tendon is becoming more common because of the fitness craze amongst the older generation. Tennis, squash and running, are the commonest activities involved. Almost half of the patients are over 35 years, and most are men.

This is a dramatic incident and the patient knows that something has snapped – they often think they have been shot, especially if there is a loud crack, or that they have been hit with a brick. After the incident, the patient can't walk properly as the calf muscles are no longer connected to the heel.

In these patients, there is no 'push off' in the normal heel-toe action in walking, but the patient can still plantar flex the ankle (weakly and not against resistance) because the tibialis posterior, toe flexors, and peroneal muscles are still working.

When you examine the patient there is no power in the plantar flexion of the foot and there is a palpable gap in the heel cord – compare with the other leg (Fig.6.1).

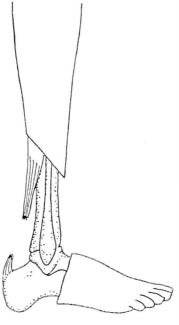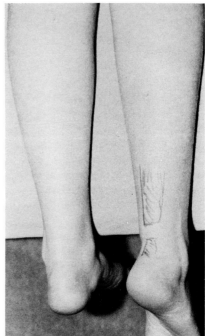

Fig. 6.1   Rupture of the tendo-achillis – you can feel the gap.

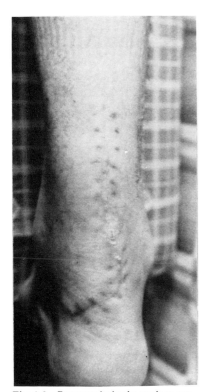

Fig. 6.2 Postoperatively, the gap has gone and the tendon works actively.

This is a clinical diagnosis and X-rays are not necessary. If they are done, they will show a gap in the soft tissue outline of the Achilles' tendon.

Operative treatment is usually necessary for complete ruptures of the tendo-achillis (Fig. 6.2). However, there are some advocates of conservative treatment by plaster immobilization in plantar flexion.

Partial ruptures can be treated by plaster immobilization **with the ankle plantar flexed 10 degrees** for four to six weeks. Crutches will be necessary during this time and of course no sport for three months after the patient comes out of plaster.

Mallet finger

This is a common problem due to rupture of the extensor mechanism of a finger at the distal insertion (Fig. 6.3).

In sport it occurs when a cricket ball or a baseball is not caught properly and the finger tip is forcibly flexed against resistance.

On the domestic front, the injury commonly occurs whilst a housewife is tucking in a bed – the mechanism is the same.

The thumb is rarely involved, but the middle, ring and little fingers are commonly injured in this way.

There are two types of anatomical lesion (Fig. 6.3b).

Fig. 6.3(a) Mallet finger – clinical picture; **(b)** the anatomical lesion; and **(c)** the X-ray picture when a piece of bone is avulsed.

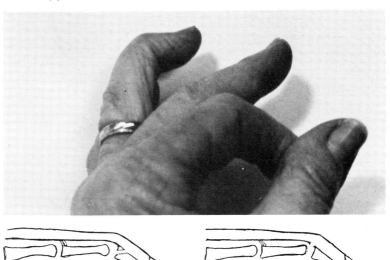

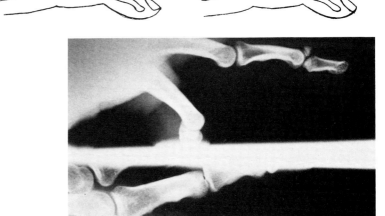

Management

Both types will respond to prolonged splinting of the finger in full extension at the distal interphalangeal joint (Fig. 6.4). **The splinting needs to be continuous for six weeks.** Most patients find this to be a real nuisance and give up during this time.

An alternative, for those who need to use their hands and cannot spare six weeks for splinting, is to insert a Kirshner wire across the joint and to bury the wire (which is bent over to prevent it wandering down the finger) in the distal pulp (Fig. 6.4). The wire is removed after the six weeks.

Fig. 6.4　Treatment of a Mallet finger can be by splintage, or a K-wire.

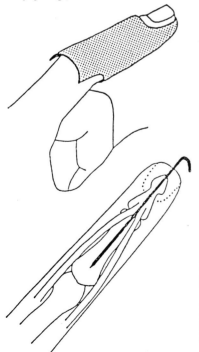

Rupture of the biceps humerus

Rupture of the long head

Your patient is typically a middle aged man, often a manual labourer who is lifting or pushing something heavy. He feels something snap just below the shoulder and has some pain in that area.

When you examine the patient he will show you that the muscle belly of the biceps muscle is **bigger than it was before the incident** (Fig. 6.5). He will also have some tenderness in the upper part of the arm and over the shoulder joint and will rapidly develop some bruising.

The tendon of the long head of the biceps has ruptured in the bicipital groove of the humerus.

Management

Although the biceps is a powerful flexor of the elbow, rupture of the long head of the biceps does not cause much weakness of this muscle, as the short head is still functioning. Repair is unnecessary and the cosmetic and functional disability should be accepted. The patient is advised that with exercise (after the initial bruising and pain have settled) the arm can be used for all work and leisure activities. A short course of physiotherapy treatment is often advisable.

Fig. 6.5　Rupture of the long head of the biceps.

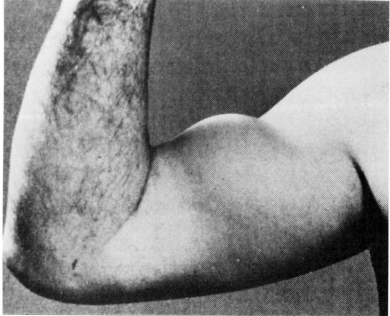

Rupture of the biceps tendon

A much rarer but more serious problem because the biceps muscle is now totally out of action. The rupture occurs at the insertion of the biceps into the neck of the radius (Fig. 6.6) – the patient feels something snap at the elbow and loses power in elbow flexion.

Clinically there is a gap, tenderness and bruising in the cubital fossa – **surgical repair is essential.**

Fig. 6.6   Rupture of the biceps tendon near its insertion.

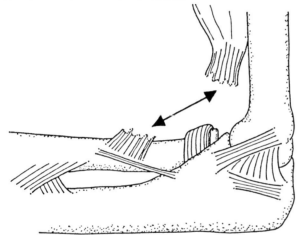

Tendon injuries in the hand

Both the flexor and extensor tendons are commonly damaged in hand injuries, and recognition and early treatment is important. **Nerves are commonly severed at the same time as the tendons are injured (Fig. 6.7).**

Fig. 6.7   A common cause of tendon and nerve damage in the hand – a sharp knife.

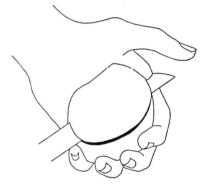

In these patients it is important to know the cause of injury and the time of injury. Obviously a recent cut with a surgically clean scalpel will be handled differently to a three day old stab wound with a fishing knife.

Now look at the wound – if any tendons are visible, see if they are partly severed (but do not poke around in the wound) and note the position and direction of the wound. **Now test the function of the tendons and nerves in the hand. All this can be done without touching the wound, by testing movement and sensation.**

Step by step:

1. Test for active movement of the distal interphalangeal (I.P.) joint in flexion (Fig. 6.8), this proves the flexor digitorum profundus is intact.

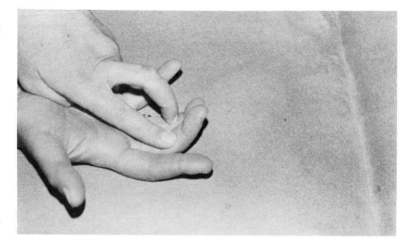

Fig. 6.8   Testing hand function – flexion of the distal interphalangeal (I-P) joint by the profundus tendon.

2. Test the flexion of each finger at the proximal interphalangeal joint (Fig. 6.9). This tests the flexor digitorum superficialis tendon.

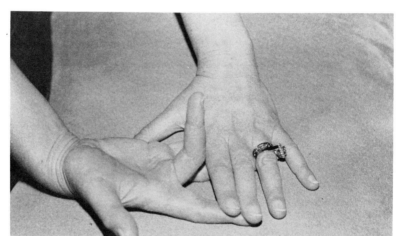

Fig. 6.9   Testing individual finger flexion by the superficialis tendon.

3. Test the thumb for active flexion and extension at the IP joint (Fig. 6.10). This will tell you if the flexor pollicus longus and the extensor pollicus longus are intact.

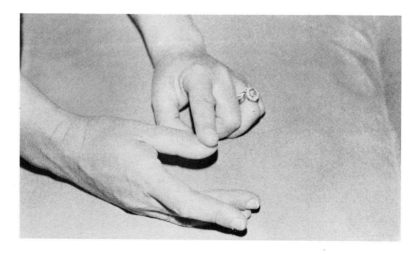

Fig. 6.10   Testing the thumb tendons, flexion, extension, abduction and adduction.

4. Test active extension both at the metacarpo-phalangeal (M.P.) joint and distally, in the fingers (Fig. 6.11). This tests the extensor mechanism proximally and distally.

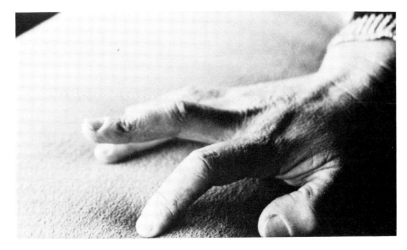

Fig. 6.11 Testing active extension of the fingers.

5. Test sensation to pin prick over the hand and fingers distal to the cut (Fig. 6.12).

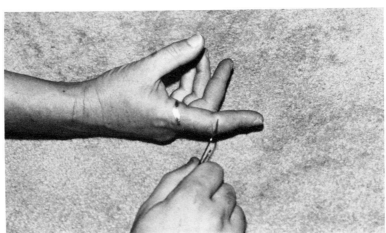

Fig. 6.12 Testing sensation, distal to the injury.

Management

You now have an accurate picture of the cause, site and extent of the injury **and the structures that have been cut.**

Primary treatment of the cut flexor tendon will vary depending on the skill that is available.

Your role in casualty will be to stop the bleeding by a pressure dressing and elevation of the hand. If there is to be immediate primary repair, that is all that is necessary.

If there is to be delayed repair, closure of the skin may be required.

Depending on the type of wound and the cause, antibiotics and tetanus prophylaxis may be indicated.

Tendon and nerve injuries at the wrist

The wrist is a crowded place, especially on the ventral aspect (Fig. 6.13) and it is hard to avoid damaging tendons and nerves in any deep injury.

Deep wounds on the ulnar border (Fig. 6.14) tend to divide the flexor carpi ulnaris, the ulnar nerve and artery, and a number of superficialis tendons to the fingers.

Deep wounds on the ventral and radial aspects of the wrist (Fig. 6.15) often divide the median nerve, the flexor carpi radialis tendon, and some of the superficialis and profundus tendons.

You will need to test the function of the flexors and extensors of the wrist, the flexors and extensors of the fingers, and the three nerves and new branches, in order to assess the effects of the nerve and tendon injury.

The testing to assess the damage is again step by step:

1. Test the tendons that move the fingers as we did in the previous section. Test both the profundus tendon moving the distal joint in active flexion and the superficialis tendon (Fig. 6.16) providing active independent flexion for each finger at the proximal interphalangeal joint.

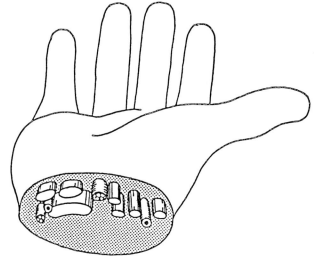

Fig. 6.13   Cross section of wrist.

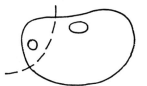

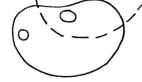

Fig. 6.14   A cut on the ulnar side of the wrist.   **Fig. 6.15**   The structures which could be damaged on the ventral surface by a penetrating wound.

Fig. 6.16   Testing flexor tendon function after a wrist injury.

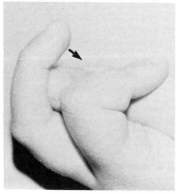

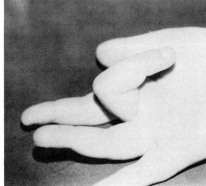

2. Test the tendons that flex the wrist by testing active flexion (Fig. 6.17) – note if there is only one group working, i.e. the ulnar or radial side.

3. Test the median nerve by testing **sensation as marked in Fig. 6.18**. The abductor pollicis brevis is the only muscle always supplied by the median nerve.

Abduct the thumb (Fig. 6.19) and ask the patient to keep it there whilst you try and push it down to the palm. The short abductor can be felt in action in the thenar eminence.

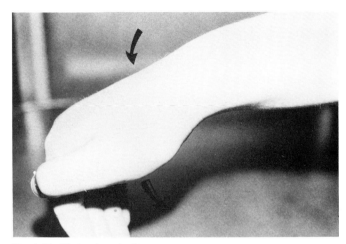

Fig. 6.17 Testing the wrist flexors.

4. Test the function of the ulnar nerve by testing the sensation in the little and half of the ring finger (Fig. 6.20) and by asking the patient to abduct the little finger (Fig. 6.21), or to adduct the thumb.

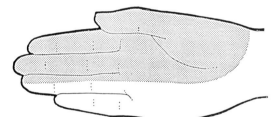

Fig. 6.18 Testing function in the median nerve – sensation.

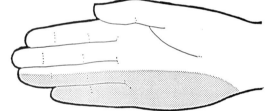

Fig. 6.20 Testing function in the ulnar nerve – sensation.

Fig. 6.19 Testing function in the median nerve – abduction of the thumb.

Fig. 6.21 Testing function in the ulnar nerve – abduction of the little finger.

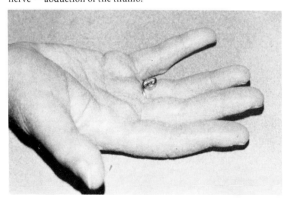

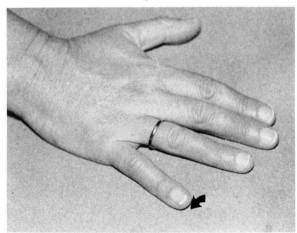

5. Loss of function in the radial nerve is tested by loss of extension of the wrist (Fig. 6.22). This of course applies to damage to the radial nerve in a high lesion, above the elbow. At the wrist, the radial nerve is purely a sensory nerve supplying a small area at the base of the thumb, on the dorsal aspect (Fig. 6.23).

6. Test the extensors as we discussed in the previous section (Figs. 6.24, 6.25 and 6.26).

There are two radial extensors of the wrist and two extensors of the index and often of the little finger. The radial nerve is often damaged in injuries to the radial side of the dorsal aspect of the wrist, as is the extensor pollicus longus (Fig. 6.24) and the extensor carpi radialis longus and brevis (Fig. 6.26).

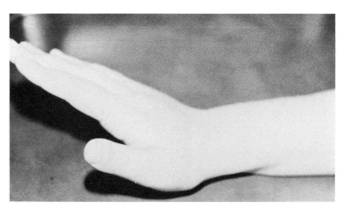

Fig. 6.22   Testing extension of the fingers.

Fig. 6.23   Testing for radial nerve − sensation.

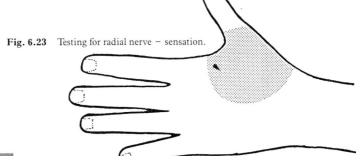

Fig. 6.24   Testing for finger extension.

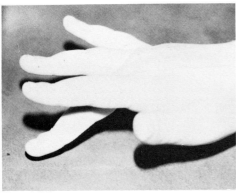

Fig. 6.25   Testing for thumb extension.

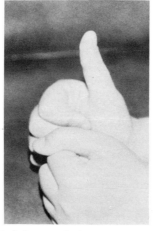

Fig. 6.26   Testing for wrist extension.

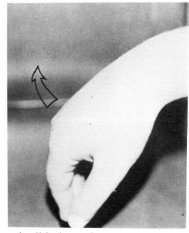

Management

All tendon and nerve damage needs to be repaired under ideal conditions with an expert doing the job. Initial treatment should include suturing the skin if there is to be some delay, otherwise a firm dressing and elevation will control the bleeding.

Naturally it is a surgical emergency if the circulation in the hand or part of the hand is compromised by damage to the ulnar and/or radial artery.

Antibiotics and tetanus prophylaxis may be necessary according to the type of wound.

CHAPTER SEVEN

The limping child

The limping child

Use the flowchart (Fig. 7.1) to help you in the investigation of the patient and refer to the following sections for more information on their early management.

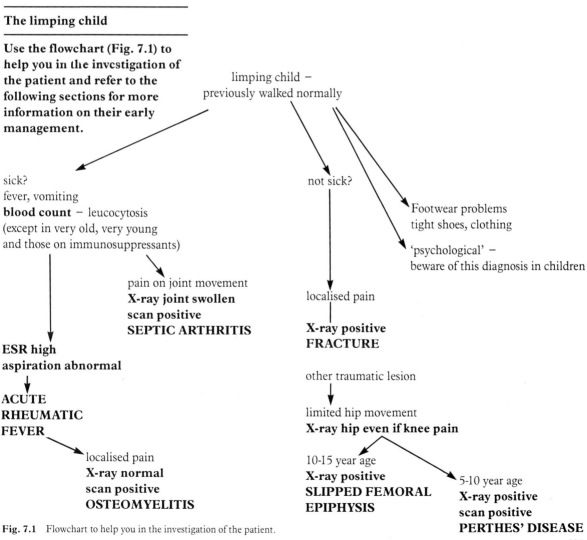

limping child –
previously walked normally

sick?
fever, vomiting
blood count – leucocytosis
(except in very old, very young
and those on immunosuppressants)

pain on joint movement
**X-ray joint swollen
scan positive
SEPTIC ARTHRITIS**

**ESR high
aspiration abnormal**

**ACUTE
RHEUMATIC
FEVER**

localised pain
**X-ray normal
scan positive
OSTEOMYELITIS**

not sick?

Footwear problems
tight shoes, clothing

'psychological' –
beware of this diagnosis in children

localised pain

**X-ray positive
FRACTURE**

other traumatic lesion

limited hip movement
X-ray hip even if knee pain

10-15 year age
**X-ray positive
SLIPPED FEMORAL
EPIPHYSIS**

5-10 year age
**X-ray positive
scan positive
PERTHES' DISEASE**

Fig. 7.1 Flowchart to help you in the investigation of the patient.

Osteomyelitis – recognition and early management

A bone infection is a serious condition – early diagnosis and correct treatment are vital factors in the prevention of complications. **The diagnosis is a clinical one, since there are no conclusive tests apart from a bone scan – which may not be readily available.**

A bone infection can be likened to a fire. It can be a sudden fierce blaze or a smouldering fire that finally bursts into flame. It can die down (under treatment) and flare up again. Osteomyelitis can be acute or chronic – acute can become chronic and chronic can become acute.

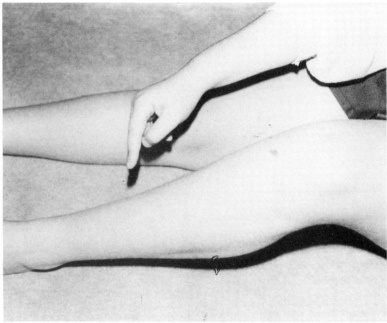

Fig. 7.2   Osteomyelitis – the child can point to the site of tenderness.

Acute osteomyelitis

This condition is mainly caused by Staphyloccus aureus and it often affects the 5-15 year age bracket. There may be a history of trauma or of skin infection, such as a boil or pimples.

The clinical picture is of an acutely ill febrile child with a painful limb and acute tenderness over the focus of infection at the end of a long bone. Swelling and redness are later signs and usually indicate abscess formation. The child can accurately point to the site of tenderness (Fig. 7.2) and usually cries when the limb is moved.

What does the X-ray show at this stage? Nothing!

As you can see from Figure 7.3, changes do not occur for about ten days. The first changes are periosteal thickening (Fig. 7.4).

Fig. 7.3   The X-ray pictures of acute osteomyelitis – nothing until day 10 and then periosteal thickening and later, day 18, bone destruction.

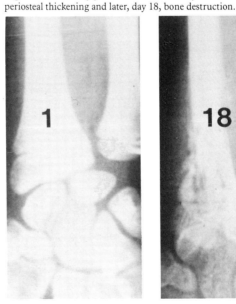
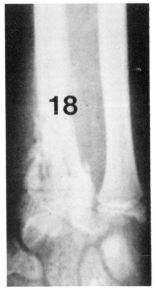
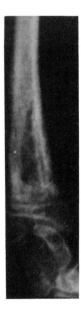

Subsequently, depending on the effectiveness of the treatment, there may be bone destruction (Fig. 7.4) and the formation of sequestra (dead bone) (Fig. 7.5). Remember this is a fight between bacteriae and the body's defences, so what happens depends on the relative strengths of the opponents.

What does the blood picture show? As with all infections, there is a leukocytosis with a shift to the left.

As this is an infection spread by the blood, there may be bacteria in the blood. Thus an early blood culture may enable you to isolate the organism and establish its sensitivity to various antibiotics within 48 hours.

Note that the physical signs are not as obvious in the very young, the very old, those on immunosuppressive drugs and those patients who have had antibiotic therapy.

A bone scan will show a focal point of increased uptake and the pooled studies will confirm this.

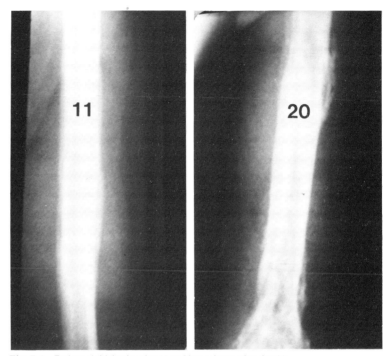

Fig. 7.4   Periosteal thickening day 11 and bone destruction day 20.

Fig. 7.5   A sequestrum in chronic osteomyelitis.

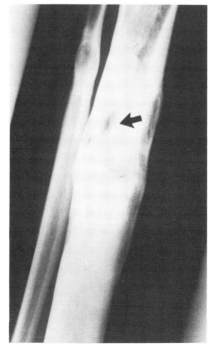

Early management

1. Make the diagnosis on the history, the presence of local tenderness, the blood picture, the normal X-ray (which would exclude a fracture) and perhaps the scan.

2. Arrange admission of the child for intensive intravenous antibiotic therapy.

3. Set up an i.v. drip and give a loading dose of antibiotic appropriate for the age and size of the child. Penicillin and Methicillin are used unless the child is allergic to penicillin. If the child is allergic to penicillin then some would use cephalosporin derivatives and others feel that there can be a cross sensitivity to cepalosporins and advise Erythromycin.

4. Splint the limb for the patient's comfort. Leave the tender area available for inspection.

5. If the condition is not resolving in 24 hours, an operation to drain any abscess and drill the bone is necessary.

Chronic osteomyelitis

In this condition there is no problem in diagnosis – the patient will tell you the diagnosis. The management of such a patient in the casualty department is clear.

If there is a flare up of a chronic infection, then you will need to order an X-ray to see if there is a sequestrum present (Figs. 7.5 and 7.6). You will also need to have a swab sent off for culture of the organisms and sensitivity to antibiotics.

Chronic osteomyelitis will not clear up with antibiotics alone if there is an abscess in the bone or a sequestrum present. The abscess (Brodie's) will need to be drained and the sequestra removed (Figs. 7.7 and 7.8).

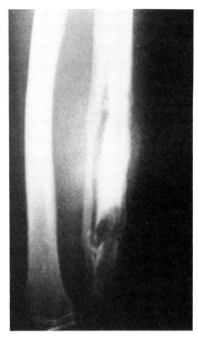

Fig. 7.6   Extensive bone destruction in chronic osteomyelitis.

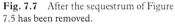

Fig. 7.7   After the sequestrum of Figure 7.5 has been removed.

Fig. 7.8   Brodie's abscess – drainage is needed.

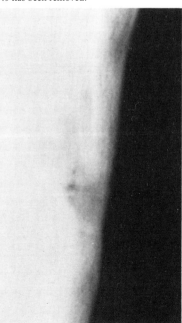

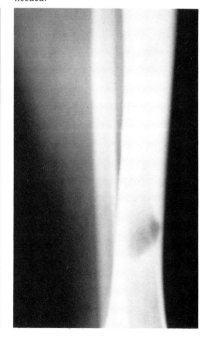

Acute septic arthritis

This is a diagnostic and treatment emergency and your role in the treatment of this condition is a *vital* one.

The condition arises either as an extension of an osteomyelitis in an adjacent bone, or as an infection in the joint following a haematogenous seeding by bacteria. It can also follow operative treatment of a knee problem, such as an arthroscopy, meniscectomy, or even aspiration.

In young babies there will be minimal signs – just a sick child with a fever (even the leukocytosis is suppressed in the very young), and a cry of pain whenever the limb is moved.

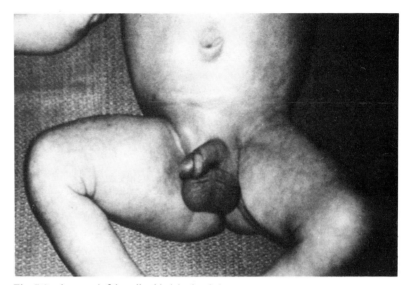

Fig. 7.9 A very painful swollen hip joint in a baby.

Fig. 7.10 The hip joint of a young baby showing distension with pus.

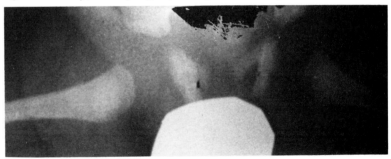

Treatment of acute septic arthritis

1. Make the diagnosis from the limited history, the painful joint (Fig. 7.9), the leukocytosis and perhaps the scan. An X-ray may be helpful in showing that the joint space is increased (Fig. 7.10).
2. Admit the child to hospital for antibiotic therapy and drainage of the joint.
3. In an adult, the joint can be aspirated under local anaesthetic and the fluid examined by the pathologists for the presence of pus cells or crystals – gout and pseudo-gout can mimic acute septic arthritis. The fluid can be cultured to isolate the organism and test its sensitivity.

4. Arrange an operation for drainage of the joint.

Articular cartilage is irreparably damaged by the presence of pus in a joint. Early diagnosis and treatment can make a real difference.

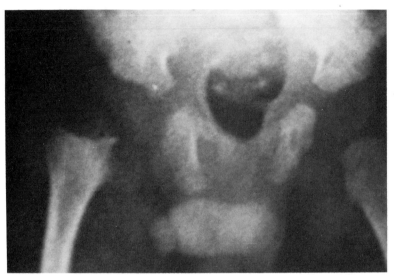

Figure 7.11 shows the distended hip on the left and the destruction of the femoral capital epiphysis.

The end result of this (so called Tom Smith) arthritis of infancy is a destroyed hip (Fig. 7.12) with a grossly shortened limb. Prevent this, by picking up these cases and treating them aggressively.

Fig. 7.11   Destruction of the femoral capital epiphysis.

Fig. 7.12   The end result of Tom Smith infective arthritis of infancy.

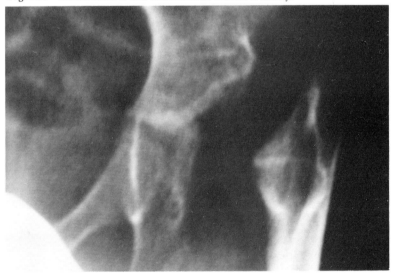

Perthes' disease (Legg – Perthes – Calvé disease)

This child will present with a limp (see Fig. 7.1) and a varying amount of pain and discomfort in the hip. There will also be a varying amount of restriction of hip movement.

X-rays in the early stage may appear normal, but the scan (Fig. 7.13) is diagnostic.

The earliest change seen on X-rays is the subchondral fracture (Fig. 7.14).

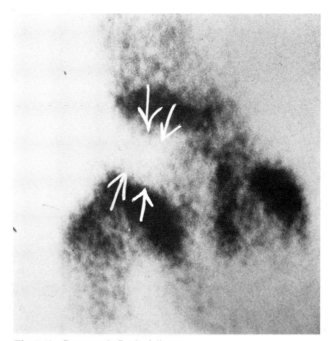

Fig. 7.13   Bone scan in Perthes' disease.

Fig. 7.14   The subchondral fracture in Perthes' disease.

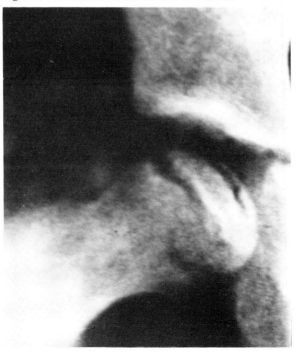

Then the epiphysis of the femoral head flattens and often fragments (Figs. 7.15 and 7.16).

Note that the condition may present in the child at a late stage with distortion of the head of the femur (Fig. 7.17).

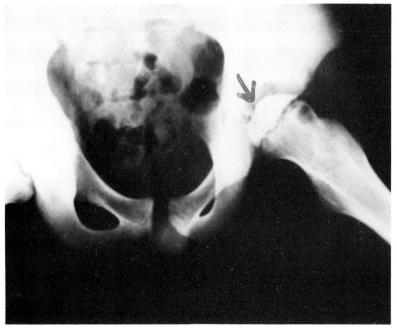

Fig. 7.15   Increased density and flattening of the femoral capital epiphysis.

Fig. 7.16   Further flattening of the epiphysis.

Fig. 7.17   The healing phase – the head is distorted.

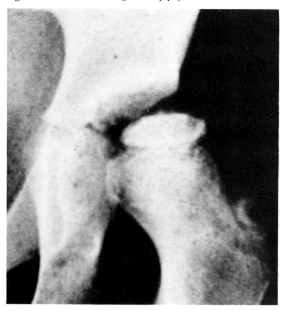

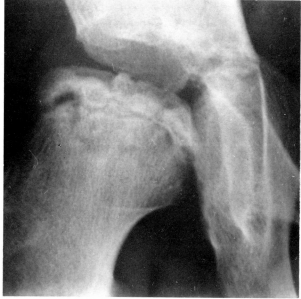

Management

Your role in the treatment is to forward the patient with their X-rays and the scan result to the orthopaedic surgeon. He will need to assess the age of the patient, the severity and stage of the disease, to try and advise the best treatment in this case. Treatment can vary from impossible, to splinting over a long time operative treatment.

Slipped upper femoral epiphysis

This condition occurs in adolescents, when the upper femoral epiphysis becomes displaced: 'like an ice cream slipping from a cone' (Figs. 7.18-7.21).

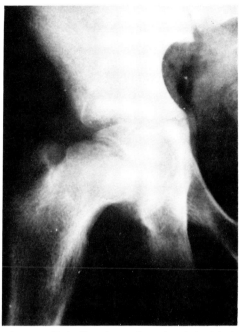

Fig. 7.18   Early slipped upper femoral capital epiphysis.

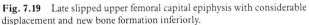

Fig. 7.19   Late slipped upper femoral capital epiphysis with considerable displacement and new bone formation inferiorly.

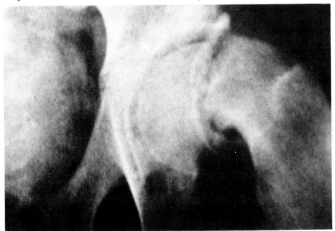

Fig. 7.20   Slipped epiphysis – the lateral view.

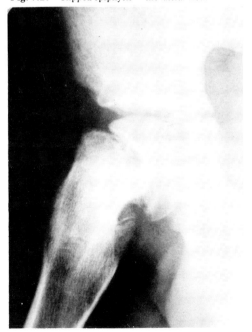

This is really a pathological fracture brought on by an abnormality of the growth plate. The patients are usually oversized, sexually underdeveloped, boys more often than girls, and generally between 10 and 15 years old.

In about 70 per cent of cases, the slip is gradual and sudden or acute in the remainder. There may be a history of trauma.

There is always limitation of movement in abduction and internal (medial) rotation.

Look at the X-rays (Fig. 7.20) and note that the ice cream has slipped in the cone — it goes inferiorly and posteriorly (Figs. 7.20 and 7.21). This child will need to be admitted to hospital and have operative treatment (Fig. 7.22) — beware of a similar but silent slip in the other hip.

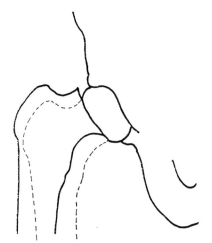

Fig. 7.21   The epiphysis slips inferiorly and posteriorly.

Fig. 7.22   The slipped epiphysis of Figure 7.20 after operative treatment.

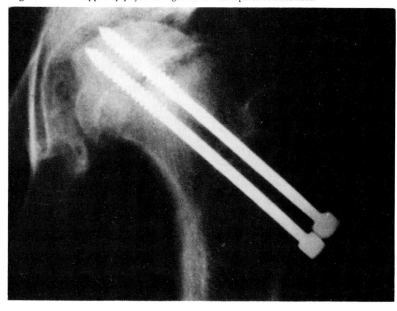

CHAPTER EIGHT

An approach to back and neck pain

'The spine is a series of bones running down your back. You sit on one end of it and your head sits on the other.'

Most housemen approach the problem of back pain by running away from it as fast as possible.

Back pain

1. *History*

(a) How long has the pain been present? Any injury or cause for pain?

(b) What type of pain?

(c) Where is the pain?

(d) Is it related to: standing, sitting, lying, bending, lifting, walking, micturition, and/or menstruation?

(e) Is it present: all day, all night, or in episodes?

(f) What makes it worse?

(g) What makes it better?

2. *Physical examination*

This must include: examination of the back movements; neurological examination in the legs; abdominal examination; and, if indicated, a pelvic examination. Note any obvious exaggerations, or inconsistencies.

3. *X-rays of the lumbar and sacral area*

These must be of good quality (Figs. 8.1 and 8.2) and include oblique views.

Fig. 8.1 The antero-posterior view of the lumbar spine.

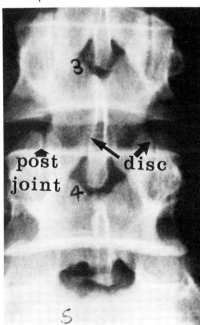

Fig. 8.2 The lateral view of the lumbar spine.

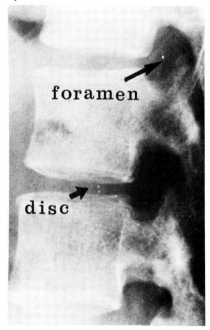

4. *Computerized tomography (C.T.)*

C. T. scanning is of great value in localizing lesions, and showing detail (Fig. 8.3).

Myelograms and *discograms* (Figs. 8.4 and 8.5) are used in the diagnosis of back pain with scitatica. It is a preoperative investigation not a general one and it has a definite morbidity. Myelography localizes the level of a lesion and indicates cord or nerve root compression (Fig. 8.4). Figure 8.6 shows the anatomy of the region. Discography gives information about a specific disc (Fig. 8.5).

Bone scanning, using radioactive material and a gamma camera will give you a good indication of any abnormal activity level in a segment of the spine. Some scans are specific, while others just indicate an abnormality.

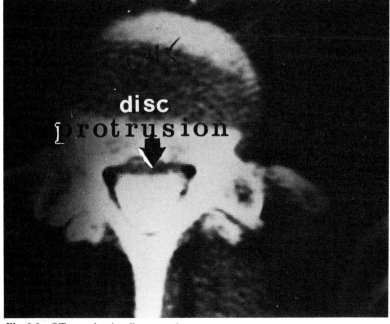

Fig. 8.3   C.T. scan showing disc protrusion.

Fig. 8.5   Discogram showing a burst L4-5 disc.

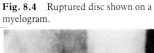

Fig. 8.4   Ruptured disc shown on a myelogram.

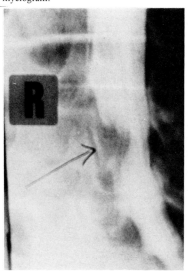

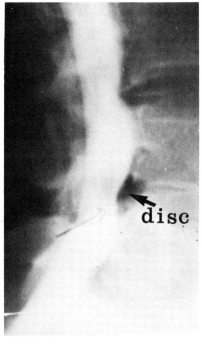

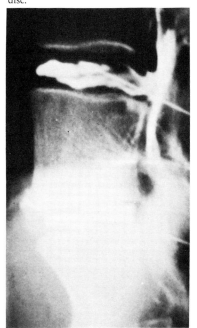

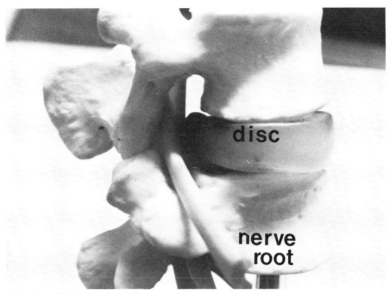

Fig. 8.6 Model showing a disc protrusion.

5. *E.m.g.*

This is a method of electrical testing for nerve function – it helps to localize the lesion.

Having taken the history, examined the patient, and having at least seen the plain X-rays; you are now in a position to diagnose and, at least, order the initial treatment of many back problems.

There are two groups of patients:

A. Those with back pain only

Reasons:

(a) Mechanical;
(b) Visceral; and
(c) Other causes.

B. Those with back pain and sciatica

Reasons:

(a) Intervertebral disc lesion; and
(b) Other causes.

Back pain only – common causes

(a) Mechanical

Trauma is a common cause of back pain and varies from bruising to fractures. The plain X-ray will distinguish the bruise from the fracture (Fig. 8.7). Bruising requires analgesics and heat, usually in the form of short wave. Fractures are dealt with in the section on *Fractures and fracture dislocations of the spine* in Chapter 3.

‘Lumbago’ and ‘fibrositis’ are non specific terms used by patients to mean pain in the lower lumbar region – usually occurring after a spell of bending and lifting. On examination, the only positive finding is some local tenderness and some muscle spasm.

X-rays are normal or show changes according to the patient's age. Treatment is rest, heat and analgesics. Most lesions settle down in a few days.

Incidentally, the term ‘fibrositis’ was introduced by Sir William Gowers in 1904.

Fig. 8.7 A crush fracture deranges the mechanics of the spine.

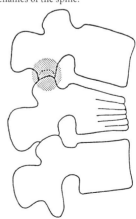

Degenerative disc disease is very common, as we all wear out steadily. In the spine, once the disc starts to degenerate, abnormal mobility occurs and then the posterior joints can become painful, especially with minor strains (Fig. 8.8a and b).

At a later stage, there is narrowing of the disc space and this is clearly visible on X-rays. When there is loss of height of the disc then there must be a strain on the posterior joints (Fig. 8.8b). This is, of course, exaggerated if the patient is overweight, has poor abdominal muscles, and/or wears high heels.

This problem may be a recurring one and the initial management will include the use of analgesics, physiotherapy, and an attempt to overcome causative factors such as obesity and job problems. Other measures, such as a few days of bed rest and traction, are occasionally necessary. If symptoms recur, some patients may be prescribed a support as well as a series of back extension exercises.

Spondylolisthesis (Figs. 8.9 and 8.10) is not uncommon and whilst it may be a chance finding on X-ray, it is often associated with back pain that recurs. The plain X-ray (Fig. 8.10) will show the lesion and it is best seen on the oblique views. The initial treatment of this lesion is as detailed in the section above; but some cases where the symptoms recur and are severe need spinal fusion. Sometimes the

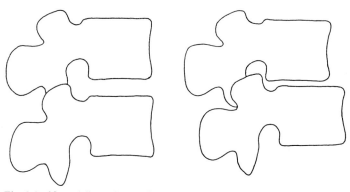

Fig. 8.8   Normal disc and worn disc with abnormal mobility.

Fig. 8.9   Spondylolisthesis.

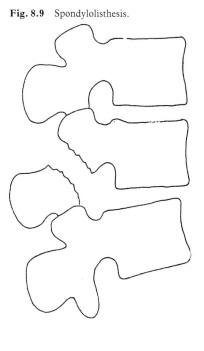

Fig. 8.10   Lateral X-ray of the lumbar spine showing spodylolisthesis with forward slip of L5 on the sacrum.

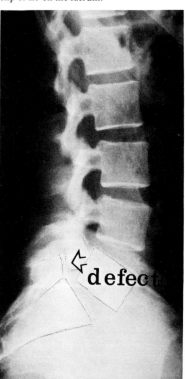

defect in the pars interarticularis is present without forward slip of the vertebrae above − the condition is then known as *spondylolysis* (Fig. 8.11).

Fig. 8.11 Spondylolysis.

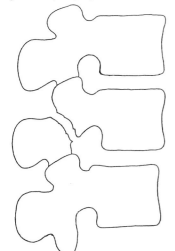

Fig. 8.12 Osteoporosis.

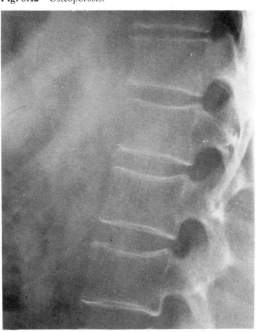

Osteoporosis, or more correctly, demineralization of the spine (Fig. 8.12) can cause pain, often due to a minor crush fracture. Demineralization occurs often in postmenopausal women and in those on steroids. Loss of density can be seen on the plain X-rays (Fig. 8.12). The lesion has to be differentiated from myeloma. Treatment will include calcium, fluoride, and sometimes hormones as well as an exercise programme.

Osteomalacia (adult rickets) is rarely due to a vitamin lack and is usually due to a failure to deposit calcium salts in normal osteoid because of renal disease or steatorrhoea. High Vitamin D and calcium supplements are needed.

(b) Visceral causes

These are not uncommon. Pelvic infections and even the use of an intra-uterine contraceptive device have been known to cause back problems. The clue to the cause lying within the pelvis will be the association of the back pain with menstruation and heavy bleeding, or abnormal bleeding.

Referral to and examination of the patient by a gynaecologist is always advisable when the symptoms are related to menstruation.

However, pain in the back during intercourse is a frequent symptom in patients with mechanical back problems.

(c) Other causes

Aneurysm of the aorta is a classical but uncommon cause of back pain (Fig. 8.13). In this case, examination of the abdomen shows the presence of a pulsatile mass and the X-rays are typical.

Fig. 8.13 Pressure effect of an aneurysm of the aorta on the spine.

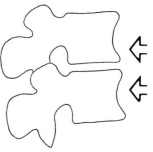

Infection is rare, but may follow discography, discectomy, or can be haematogenous. The disc space on the X-ray shows involvement of the adjacent vertebral bodies (Fig. 8.14a, b and c).

Pyogenic infection is usually due to a staphyloccocal infection and occurs in adults. About 25 per cent of the patients are diabetics; and another group, usually with gram negative infections, are the drug addicts.

Backache is the presenting symptom, and the patient may not have fever or other constitutional symptoms until an abscess forms. Therefore this can be a hard diagnosis to make. Spinal movements and jarring cause severe pain, but early X-rays do not show changes and it can be several weeks before narrowing and vertebral erosion take place (Fig. 8.14b). The diagnosis is made on the severe unremitting pain, rigid back and raised erythrocte sedimentation rate (ESR). Treatment will include: hospitalization; isolation of the organism; drainage of any abscess; and the surgical removal of dead bone.

Tuberculous infection is different in that it is very insidious – it is always secondary to tuberculosis elsewhere. X-rays show involvement of a vertebral body usually in the thoracic or upper lumbar region and the disc is relatively resistant to destruction – they may also show a psoas abscess. Back pain is a common presenting sympton, but there are often many systemic symptoms. It may be hard to distinguish tuberculous and pyogenic infection without aspiration and culture.

Neoplasm as secondary deposits in the spine can cause back pain. Sources of the primary neoplasm are lung, breast, prostate, and more rarely kidney or thyroid. As with many neoplasms, the appearance of the secondary lesion may be the first presentation of the malignancy. In this case there is no history, but the alert doctor will have this lesion in mind when examining the older age group. For example, the silver hair of a man in his sixties, who has nocturia and back pain, will always remind you to do a rectal examination to exclude carcinoma of the prostate.

Fig. 8.14a Infection in a disc space. **b** X-ray of early tuberculous infection.   **c** X-ray of late tuberculous infection.

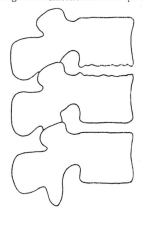
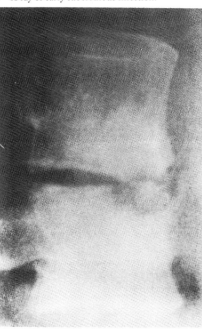
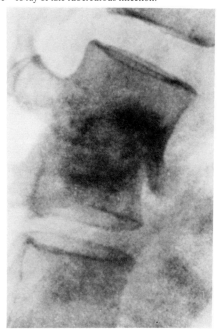

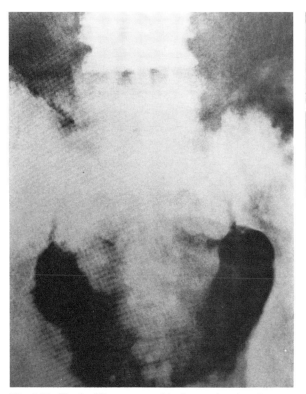 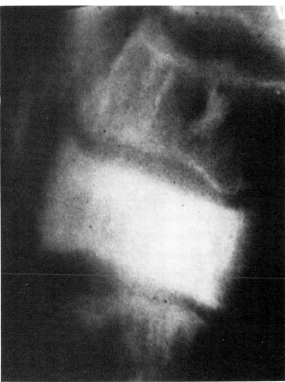

Fig. 8.15   Vertebra Nigrans – osteoblastic secondary deposits.

With a secondary deposit, the disc is spared and there is usually collapse and destruction of the vertebral body. However, some deposits are osteoblastic and give rise to a very dense vertebral body – vertebra nigrans (Fig. 8.15).

In the antero-posterior X-rays of the spine, one of the pedicles is commonly destroyed giving the so called 'winking owl' sign (Fig. 8.16).

Bone scans will show increased uptake in the areas of secondary deposits.

Fig. 8.16   The 'winking owl' sign – destruction of a pedicle.

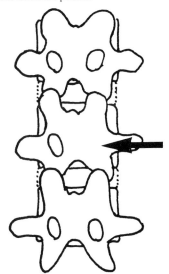

Myeloma is the most common primary malignant tumour (Fig. 8.17).

There is usually a history of backache, weakness and weight loss. A pathological fracture may occur. The sedimentation rate is always raised and Bence Jones Protein may be present in the urine in 50 per cent of cases.

X-rays show a lytic lesion in the localized form (Fig. 8.18) and diffuse demineralization in the diffuse form.

Discitis is a benign condition occurring in children. Associated with the back pain is a refusal to walk. As the condition develops, there is some muscle spasm and some localized tenderness.

This condition needs to be distinguished from vertebral osteomyelitis, and this is best done by investigation in hospital.

The treatment of this condition is rest and support. Fortunately it resolves and seems to leave no problems.

Compensation claims make the assessment of patients difficult and sometimes impossible. A clever patient can usually get medical support for his or her claim. Early in the compensation game most patients do not know their anatomy well and are inconsistent. One good test is to compare the amount of spinal movement that they will carry out bending forward, with the movement they carry out whilst on a couch when you ask them casually to sit up, lean forward, and finally to grasp their foot.

The patient who has been working at two jobs to make extra

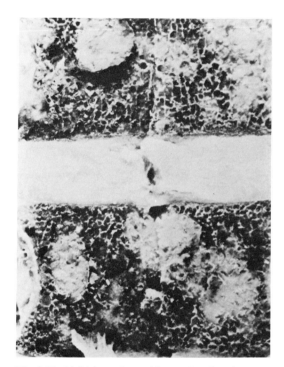

Fig. 8.17   Multiple myeloma with secondary deposits in the spine.

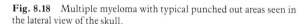

Fig. 8.18   Multiple myeloma with typical punched out areas seen in the lateral view of the skull.

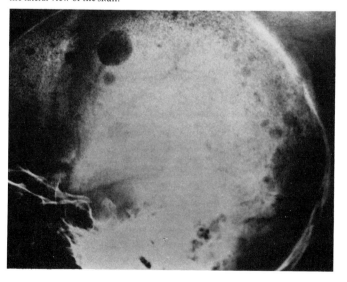

money and is injured may not be able to face the situation again, and will use the injury and its apparent failure to get better to avoid going back.

On the domestic front, a persistent back problem (real or imagined) can be a powerful weapon in an unsatisfactory marriage.

The more common causes of backache with sciatica

(a) Acute rupture of an intervertebral disc (Fig. 8.19)

This is the most common cause of backache with sciatica. Usually, there is a history of injury, often of lifting whilst bent forward. However, in many patients there is just a bending incident, such as bending over to tie shoelaces or getting up from a lounge chair.

Pain in the back followed by leg pain, which is severe and stabbing and goes down the leg often to the ankle, are common pain patterns. There may also be numbness in the distribution of the affected nerve root.

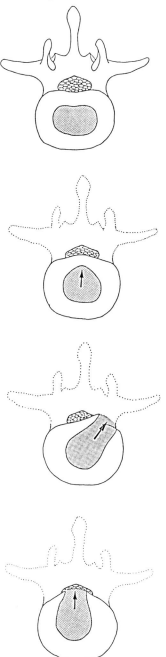

Fig. 8.19   The anatomy of a disc rupture: normal, mild midline bulge, lateral rupture, and midline rupture.

Numbness and paraesthesia over the lateral side of the foot and the sole suggest that the S1 nerve root (Fig. 8.20) is affected; and numbness over the anteriomedial aspect of the leg implies an L5 lesion (Fig. 8.21).

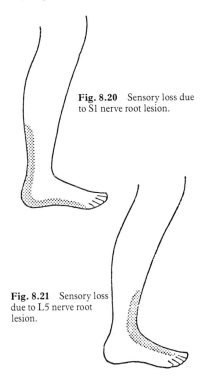

Fig. 8.20   Sensory loss due to S1 nerve root lesion.

Fig. 8.21   Sensory loss due to L5 nerve root lesion.

The patient is in severe pain and the pain is made worse by bending, stooping, sneezing and straining; there is muscle spasm and usually the patient leans towards the side that is painful – the lean worsens as the patient flexes the spine; and all movement is limited, flexion especially. Straight leg raising is limited to 20-30 degrees and causes intense sciatic pain.

There can be loss of ankle jerk, loss of sensation as mentioned, and weakness in dorsi or plantar flexion of the ankle.

This is the broad picture of a ruptured intervertebral disc. The lesion varies in severity and there is a great deal of variation in patients' ability to stand pain. Add to this the question of compensation and you can see how difficult it can be to decide how much trouble a patient has.

The patient with a severe disc lesion needs to be admitted to hospital for bed rest, traction and analgesics (see Fig. 8.22).   8.23).

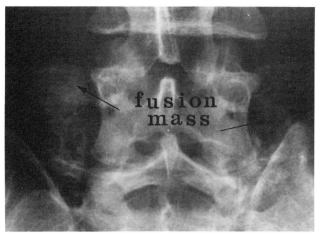

Fig. 8.22 Flowchart for the treatment of intervertebral disc lesion – rupture

Fig. 8.23 Antero-posterior view six months after a spinal fusion, showing the fusion mass.

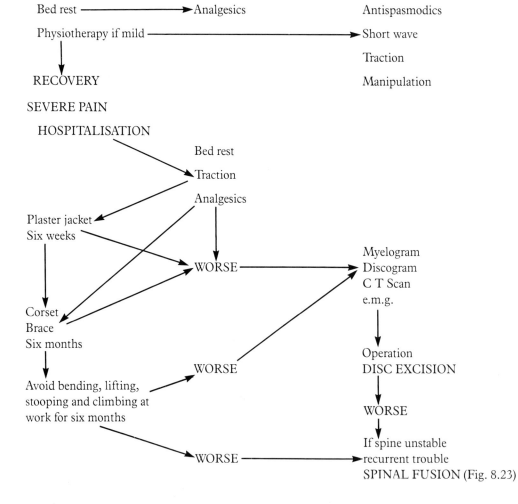

MILD PAIN

Bed rest ⟶ Analgesics   Antispasmodics

Physiotherapy if mild ⟶ Short wave

                                                 Traction

RECOVERY   Manipulation

SEVERE PAIN

  HOSPITALISATION

                        Bed rest

                        Traction

                        Analgesics

Plaster jacket
Six weeks

                        WORSE ⟶ Myelogram
                                        Discogram
                                        C T Scan
                                        e.m.g.

Corset
Brace
Six months

                        WORSE   Operation
                                                 DISC EXCISION

Avoid bending, lifting,
stooping and climbing at   WORSE
work for six months

                        WORSE ⟶ If spine unstable
                                        recurrent trouble
                                        SPINAL FUSION (Fig. 8.23)

(b) Degenerative disc disease with referred pain

This condition, in which the patient has back pain and pain referred to the buttock or pain of an aching type that goes down the leg, is very common. The patient often has multiple attacks of this type of pain occurring without warning but usually associated with a minor bending and lifting incident.

X-rays often show degenerative changes at multiple levels and the most likely cause of the pain is the posterior joints.

Acute episodes need to be managed with a combination of rest, bed rest on a hard surface, physiotherapy, analgesics and a back re-education programme. Manipulation is also of value, but should only be done if:

1. The patient is relatively young and fit;

2. There is no evidence of nerve root pressure;

3. There are no abnormal neurological signs; and

4. X-rays exclude tumour, infection and demineralization.

Some manipulative techniques are shown in Figure 8.24a.

A lot of patients who have relatively weak abdominal muscles, benefit from a programme of exercise which strengthens these and the spinal extensors (Fig. 8.24b). A support is also of value in this type of patient, but must be used in conjunction with the exercises.

Spinal metastases or pelvic tumours that involve the lumbar nerve roots can cause back pain and sciatica. There is usually enough other evidence on examination or on the X-rays to suspect such a lesion. A bone scan will indicate areas of abnormal uptake, and computerized tomography will demonstrate the lesion.

Fig. 8.24(a)   Some manipulative techniques:

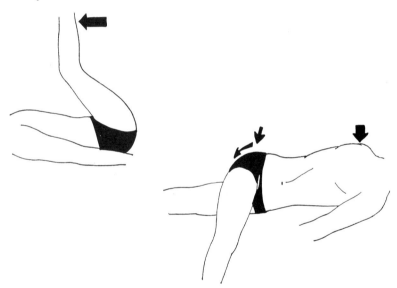

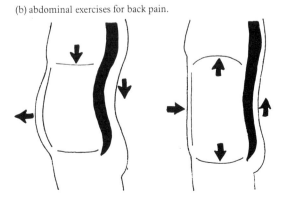

(b) abdominal exercises for back pain.

Neck pain

Neck pain may arise from the 'mechanical' elements of the spine; local viscera, such as the pharynx, larynx, oesophagus; or be referred vascular pain (cardiac or carotid).

You will need to use the following to help reach a diagnosis and plan treatment:

1. *History*
   (a) Any injury past or present?
   (b) When did the pain start?
   (c) What type of pain?
   (d) Where is the site of the pain, its spread and pattern?
   (e) What makes it better?
   (f) What makes it worse?
   (g) Is there any weakness or loss of power in the limbs?
   (h) Are there any sensory symptoms?
   (i) Is there pain on neck movement or shoulder movement?
   (j) Is there pain on exercise?

2. *Physical examination*
This will include: palpation over the cervical spinous processes and the anterior aspect of the neck, to note any tenderness or mass; movement of the neck in flexion, extension, lateral flexion and rotation (Fig. 8.25a).

Shoulder movement must also be tested and power, sensation and reflexes in all four limbs (Fig. 8.25b).

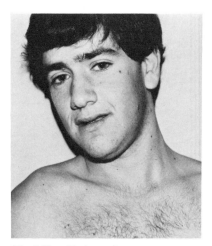
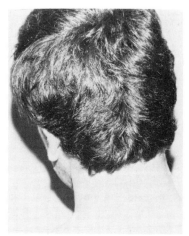

Fig. 8.25a   Testing neck movements

(b)   Testing for neurological signs in the limbs

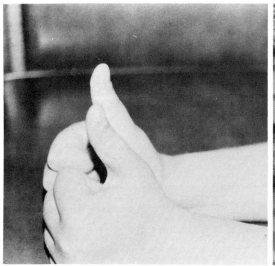
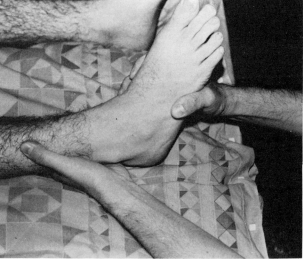

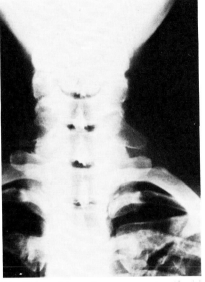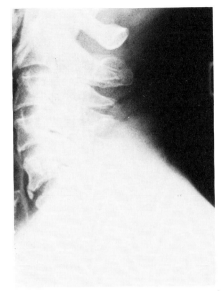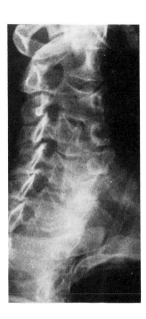

(c)   X-rays of the neck: antero-posterior, lateral and oblique films.

3. *X-ray examination*
This must include the whole of the cervical spine including oblique views, so that the intervertebral foramina can be seen and any encroachment assessed (Fig. 8.25c).

4. *Computerized axial tomography (C.T.)*
C.T. is of value in localizing and assessing the extent of a lesion at a particular level. It is a non-invasive X-ray examination.

Cervical *myelograms* and *discograms* will localize disc pathology, but are becoming less important as C.T. scanning improves.

5. *Electrocardiographs* and stress tests may be helpful in those patients with pain that may be of cardiac origin.

Common causes of neck pain

Mechanical causes

Trauma
See the section on *Fracture and fracture dislocations of the spine* – Cervical vertebrae in Chapter 3.

Acute cervical strain

This is probably what happens in the so called 'whiplash' injury common in motor vehicle accidents.

The patient presents in casualty with a history of a motor vehicle accident. There is pain and spasm with loss of some movements of the cervical spine.

There will be no loss of power or sensation in the limbs and the X-rays will be normal or show loss of the usual cervical lordosis (Fig. 8.26). (There may be some degenerative changes in the older patient.)

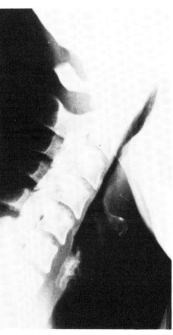

Fig. 8.26   Loss of lordosis in lateral X-ray of the cervical spine.

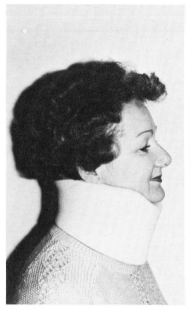

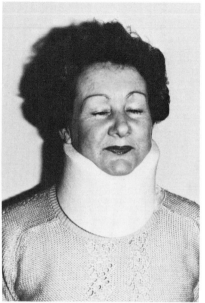

Fig. 8.27 Soft collar to rest the painful neck.

Initial treatment will depend on the amount of pain the patient is suffering and the presence of other injuries – it may suffice to apply a soft collar (Fig. 8.27) and to give the patient analgesics, but if the pain is severe it may be better to admit the patient to hospital.

Physiotherapy, in the form of short wave and mechanical traction, may be of value although this tends to be used after the first week of rest in a collar.

Persistent severe pain or the development of neurological signs must make you suspect an undetected fracture. In this case, further X-rays should always be taken.

Acute disc prolapse

This is much less common than in the lumbar region, but it presents in much the same way. There is usually a history of a provocative incident followed by neck pain and radicular pain that is severe.

There are often neurological signs present, such as weakness of the deltoid and biceps, loss of the biceps reflex and sensory loss around the base of the thumb in a C5-C6 disc lesion – this is due to compression of the C6 nerve root.

Compression of the C7 nerve root at the next most common site, the C6-C7 level, gives a different clinical picture – weakness of the triceps and diminished or absent triceps reflex with sensory changes over the index and middle fingers.

Management. These patients require to be in hospital, and will need strong analgesics. Intermittent traction through a head halter (Fig. 8.28) is of value and most patients find it best to put the traction on for a few hours and then have a rest. If the lesion fails to settle, then operative treatment may be necessary.

Fig. 8.28 Traction device for cervical traction.

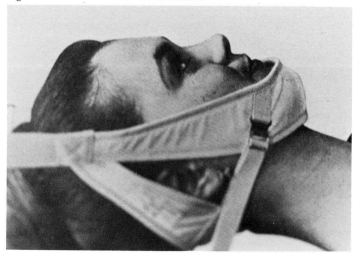

Degenerative joint disease in the cervical spine

This is common and is a common cause of both neck pain and referred pain to the shoulder and upper limb. Degenerative changes are apparent in both the discs and in the posterior joints on the X-rays (Fig. 8.29). The amount of degenerative change bears no direct relationship to the amount of pain that the patient suffers, but the neck that has degenerative changes is much more likely to suffer from acute injury with even minor trauma.

Usually the patient is middle aged and complains of pain in the neck and difficulty in turning the head, such as when reversing the car. Pain is often referred to the shoulder or even further down the arm. Depending on which segments are involved, there may be symptoms of nerve root irritation, with pain going down the outer side of the arm and, in C5-6 lesions, numbness around the base of the thumb.

Treatment of the problem includes the judicious use of a collar (Fig. 8.30), with physiotherapy in the form of short wave or traction and manipulation of the neck with or without anaesthesia. Operative treatment may be necessary for chronic unresolved lesions, and in some cases, C.T. scans or discograms are necessary to localize the lesions.

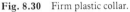
Fig. 8.30 Firm plastic collar.

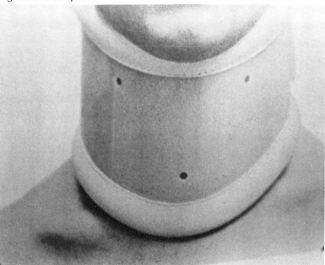

Fig. 8.29 Degenerative changes seen on the lateral view of the cervical spine.

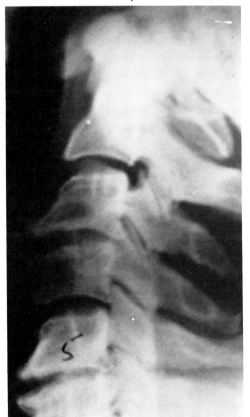

The rarer mechanical causes of neck and arm pain

This is not an exhaustive list but you should always keep in mind the possibility of:

(a) A secondary malignant lesion in the cervical vertebrae;

(b) An infective lesion in the cervical vertebrae or even in the epidural space;

(c) A neoplasm of the spinal cord; and

(d) An apical lung tumour (Pancoast tumour) causing pressure on the brachial plexus.

Malignant lesions show up on scanning (Fig. 8.31).

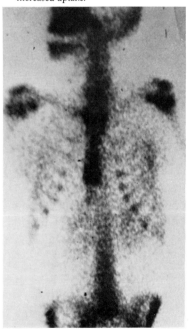

Fig. 8.31 Scan showing secondary deposits – increased uptake.

Shoulder lesions, such as a supraspinatus lesion, can have pain that radiates to the neck and down the arm. In the history, the keypoint is that the patient has pain on shoulder movement and not on neck movement. In addition, there should be no sensory symptoms in a shoulder lesion.

Examination of such a patient generally shows restriction of movement of the shoulder with pain (Fig. 8.32) and a free range of neck movement without neurological abnormalities.

Occasionally a patient will have both **a mild neck and shoulder problem at the same time.**

Cervical rib compression of the brachial plexus is not nearly as fashionable a diagnosis as it was a few years ago. Generally the patient has little or no neck pain but has radicular pain; some weakness or clumsiness; and perhaps some

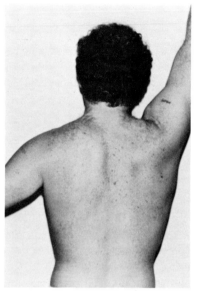

Fig. 8.32 Pain and restriction of shoulder movement.

vascular signs, such as blueness in the hand. Figure 8.33 shows a small cervical rib which was symptomless and found on another examination.

Fig. 8.33 Small cervical rib.

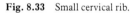

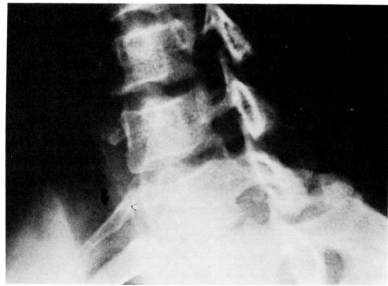

CHAPTER NINE

Knee and ankle injuries. Arm and shoulder pain

Acute knee injuries

Fractures of the distal end of the
femur and fractures of the upper
end of the tibia do involve the knee
joint and are dealt with in Chapter
4.

Knee injuries are common in
sport as well as in other activities
and you will see many in the
casualty department.

Assessment

To assess the injured knee you will
need to:

1. **Take a careful history**
Try and find out what actually
happened to the knee. Was it a
twisting injury, a straight valgus, or
varus strain or a direct blow?

2. **Examine the knee**
This can be difficult and
unrewarding in an acutely injured,
and therefore acutely painful, knee.
If it is possible, you should carefully
palpate the knee and find the tender
areas. Then put the knee through a
range of movement (Figs. 9.1 and
9.2) and test the medial, lateral and
cruciate ligaments (Figs. 9.3 and
9.4).

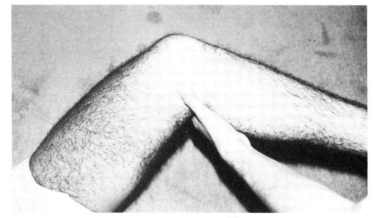

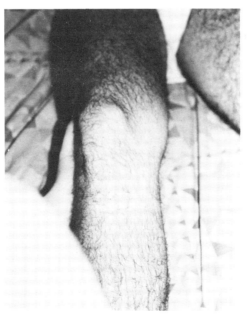

Fig. 9.1 Testing knee movement.

Fig. 9.2 Testing knee movement.

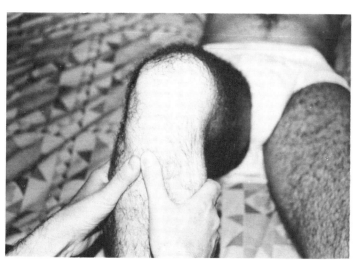

Fig. 9.3 Testing cruciate ligaments.

Fig. 9.4 Testing medial ligament.

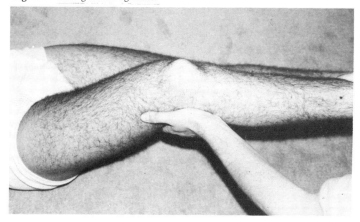

3. **X-ray the knee** including, if indicated, stress views to see if there is any instability (Fig. 9.5).

In many patients the above examination is not possible as they are in too much pain. If this is the case then the following is suggested.

1. If there is a gross haemarthrosis with a tense and very tender knee, then admit the patient and arrange an orthopaedic consultation. The patient will probably need an aspiration of the knee or, as is more commonly done these days, an examination of the

Fig. 9.5 Stress X-rays of medial and lateral sides of knee.

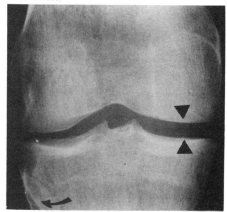

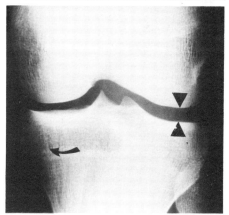

knee under anaesthesia followed by an arthroscopic assessment of the knee − after the joint has been washed out through the arthroscope.

2. If the knee is not grossly swollen and the X-ray shows no definite lesion, but the knee is too painful to examine properly, then apply a backslab and give the patient crutches and some analgesics. An alternative to a backslab is a multilayered Robert Jones bandage, in which at least four alternate layers of cotton wool and crepe bandage are applied. The patient is instructed to rest with the leg elevated and is then seen in one week − it is then possible to examine the knee thoroughly.

Ruptured ligaments

These are common injuries due to: a valgus strain in the case of the medial ligament; and a varus strain in the case of the lateral ligament. The ligaments are shown in Figures 9.6 and 9.7.

In pure ligament injuries, there is not much swelling in the joint as the injury is extra-synovial and therefore outside the joint.

Stressing of the ligaments during the examination and localized tenderness are key points in the diagnosis. Stress X-rays can be of value. If there is any doubt, then the knee should be examined under an anaesthetic.

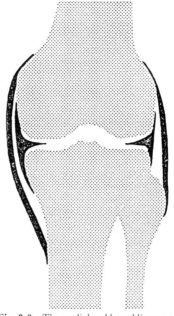

Fig. 9.6 The medial and lateral ligaments and menisci.

Fig. 9.7 View from above of the menisci and cruciate ligaments.

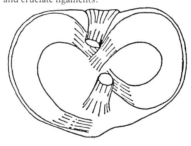

Fig. 9.8 Arthroscopic view of a torn meniscus.

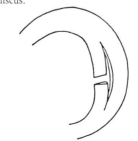

Management

Complete ruptures of the medial or lateral ligaments should be surgically repaired to obtain the best results. The ligament is often curled in at the point of rupture and therefore will not heal strongly. Repair should be carried out within the first week if possible. After operation, the patient will be in plaster for six weeks and during this time, care should be taken to keep the quadriceps strong.

Incomplete ruptures of the ligaments − where there is just a little springing − should be treated with the knee in a plaster cylinder for six weeks. During this time, the patient should carry out quadriceps exercises. See Chapter 4 for details of the application of a plaster cylinder.

Meniscus injuries

There is usually a clear history of a twisting injury with the knee partially flexed and weight bearing. The patient knows something has happened, as there is acute pain over the medial joint line (or lateral joint line in the case of a lateral meniscus injury).

The knee swells quickly, often locks and catches because **part of the meniscus catches between the condyles (Fig. 9.8).** Another common symptom, is a feeling that something is moving or clicking in the knee.

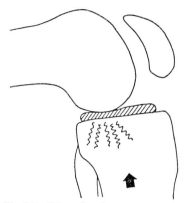

Fig. 9.9   Pain and tenderness over a torn meniscus on rotation of the knee whilst bearing weight.

When you examine the knee, you will note the acute tenderness, swelling, the lack of full extension and the pain on forced flexion of the knee (Fig. 9.9). An X-ray should be arranged to exclude bony injury or the presence of a loose body.

Often the patient limps home and the knee gradually settles down over a few weeks, only to cause trouble again when the now torn meniscus catches between the tibia and the femur.

Occasionally, the meniscus is completely split and then it may enclose the femoral condyle like a 'bucket handle' (Fig. 9.10). The knee is then locked or 'stuck' in a partially flexed position.

Fig. 9.10   Arthroscopic view of bucket handle tear of a meniscus.

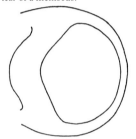

Sometimes the knee will settle down, especially if the tear is a small one, and there will be no trouble until there is a further twisting incident.

A torn meniscus is almost certainly present in a knee if:

1. There is a history of a twisting injury followed by swelling;

2. There is a localized tenderness over the joint line;

3. There is loss of full extension; and

4. There is pain and perhaps **a click on rotation of the knee, whilst weight bearing** (Fig. 9.11).

Fig. 9.11   Testing the knee by rotation whilst weight bearing.

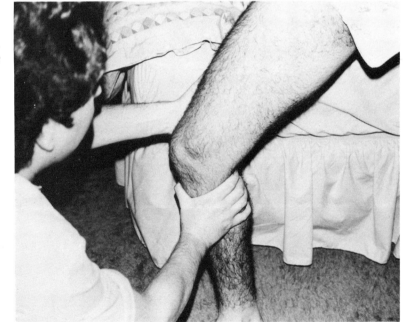

Management

Once the diagnosis of a torn meniscus is made, operative treatment is indicated.

Nowadays the diagnosis is confirmed and treatment is carried out, through the arthroscope rather than through open arthrotomy.

Arthrography (Fig. 9.12a) of the knee is of value in making the diagnosis but still leaves the patient with the lesion for treatment. Arthroscopy gives the competent arthroscopist the opportunity to confirm the diagnosis and carry out the removal of the torn meniscal fragment at the same time (Fig. 9.12b).

Fig. 9.12a Arthrogram showing a torn meniscus.
b Arthroscopic view of the meniscus in Figure 9.12a.

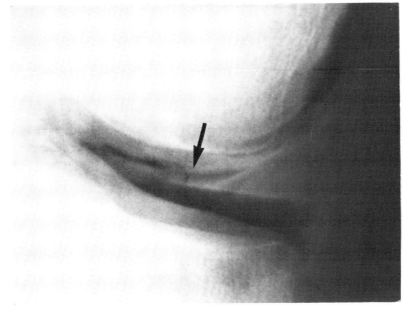

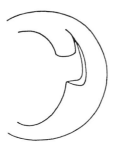

Combined meniscal and ligament lesions

Unfortunately some injuries to the knee are so severe that they tear not only the ligaments but also the capsule and meniscus.

These patients have a clear history of major trauma, have severe pain and gross swelling of the knee. There is also obvious instability as a result of the ligament damage.

Admit this patient to hospital, if it is possible, as they will require major reconstructive surgery, and the sooner this is done (within reason) the better.

If the patient insists on going home, immobilize him in a plaster slab and provide him with crutches. Arrange for the patient to be seen by an orthopaedic surgeon as soon as possible.

Ankle injuries – fractures and ligament lesions

These injuries are usually clinically obvious but an X-ray should be ordered. **Fractures** around the ankle are dealt with in Chapter 4.

Inversion injuries or 'going over on the ankle' are frequent occurrences, especially amongst ladies with high heeled shoes (Fig. 9.13).

Fig. 9.13   Inversion injury – going over on the ankle.

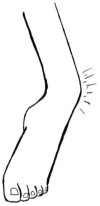

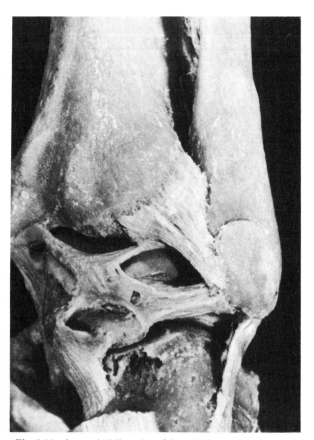

Fig. 9.14   Anatomical dissection of the ankle ligaments.

Apart from fractures, the common injury around the ankle is a **partial or complete tear of the lateral ligament**. Figure 9.14 shows an anatomical dissection of the ankle ligaments.

Clinically the pain and swelling are localized below and distal to the lateral malleolus and there is protective spasm and pain on attempted inversion (Fig. 9.15).

Fig. 9.15   Testing the lateral ligament of the ankle.

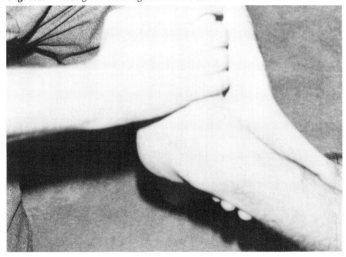

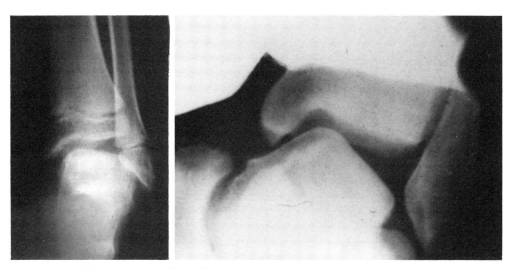

Fig. 9.16 Stress X-rays showing lateral instability.

If a complete rupture is suspected – from the history, physical examination and stress X-rays (Fig. 9.16) – then, in my view, operative repair should be undertaken. There are those who claim equally good results from conservative management.

However, there is often a partial tear of the ligament and then a regimen of protection, support and exercise without weight bearing, are advised for a few weeks. Physiotherapy in the form of heat and rotatory exercises will help the lesion resolve. Apply a firm crepe bandage supporting the injured ligament.

Chronic lateral ligament insufficiency is usually present in the patient who goes over on the ankle recurrently without sufficient reason. Stress X-rays will show talar tilt on forced inversion. Operative repair or reinforcement is indicated (Fig. 9.17). Most operations involve the use of the peroneus brevis tendon as a substitute ligament.

Medial ligament. An eversion injury can cause an isolated injury to the medial ligament of the ankle, but these injuries are rare as there tends to be a fracture of the lateral malleolus associated with the ligament injury (Fig. 9.18).

This combined injury is dealt with in the section on ankle fractures in Chapter 4. Isolated injuries require similar treatment to lateral ligament lesions.

Fig. 9.18 Medial ligament rupture associated with a fractured lateral malleolus.

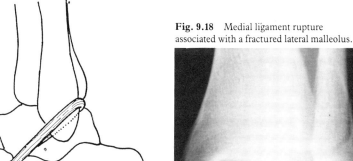

Fig. 9.17 One of the many reconstructive procedures for lateral instability.

Shoulder injuries and shoulder pain

Fractures involving the shoulder joint are dealt with in Chapter 3.

Dislocations of the shoulder are dealt with in Chapter 5.

Rupture of the long head of the biceps is dealt with in Chapter 6.

Supraspinatus lesions – lesions of the rotator cuff

Four types of lesion are possible:

1. Tearing of the capsule occurs as part of a degenerative process and the role of the injury can be fairly minor. The injury occurs as a result of lifting a weight or protecting oneself from a fall. Acute pain is referred to the deltoid insertion, and the patient is unable to initiate abduction (Fig. 9.19a).

Partial tears can recover partially, fully, or develop into a 'frozen shoulder'.

Partial tears can be distinguished from complete ones by testing movement before and after the injection of local anaesthetic into the shoulder (Fig. 9.19b, c and d).

In partial lesions the patient can then abduct the shoulder (Fig. 9.19d).

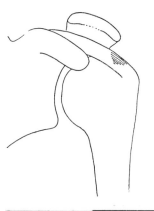

Fig. 9.19   Partial tear of the supraspinatus – movement before and after an injection of local anaesthetic.

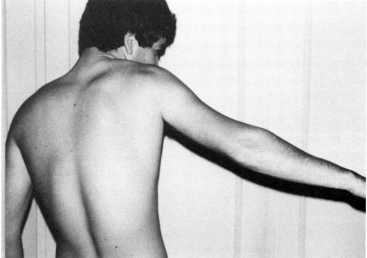

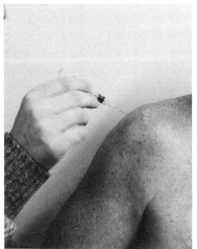

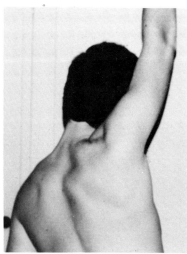

In complete lesions it is not possible to abduct the shoulder (Fig. 9.20) when the shoulder is abducted the deltoid can hold it in the abducted position. Complete lesions are very rare – some say they should be repaired surgically, but this is not essential as over a period of months abduction is restored naturally.

2. Acute tendonitis – acute calcification. This is a reaction to minor trauma – or even overuse of the shoulder – in an area of local degeneration. There is acute pain and swelling in the shoulder, the pain varying from severe to agonising (you will not be allowed to touch or move the shoulder, it is too painful).

If the patient can tolerate the pain, the lesion will settle down over about one week – usually they require your help.

Order an X-ray to show if acute calcification (Fig. 9.21) is the cause.

When acute calcification is diagnosed (Fig. 9.21), inject some hydrocortisone and local anaesthetic into the tender area. **The patient may require admission to hospital for strong analgesics.**

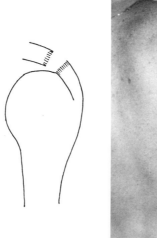
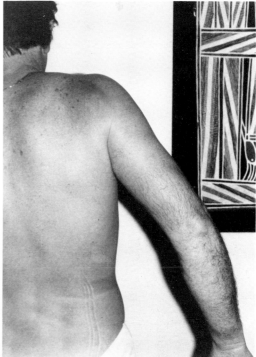

Fig. 9.20   Complete tear of the rotator cuff – inability to abduct the shoulder.

Fig. 9.21   Calcification in the supraspinatus.

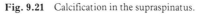
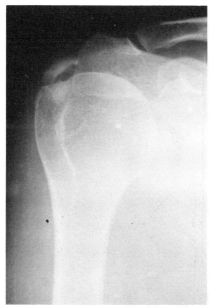

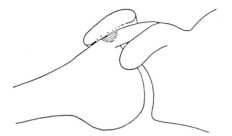

Fig. 9.22   The reason for the painful arc of abduction, i.e. the lesion rubs on the roof of the shoulder.

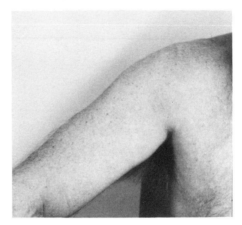

Fig. 9.23   The start of the painful arc of abduction.

3. Chronic tendonitis. This lesion is associated with a larger area of degenerative capsule and perhaps some minor trauma or overuse.

Classically, there is a painful arc of abduction of the shoulder due to the impingement of the pathological area of capsule against the 'roof of the shoulder' and this occurs between 80 and 120 degrees of abduction (Figs. 9.22 and 9.33), usually in a patient of 45 to 60 years old. The symptoms come on gradually.

Treatment of the painful arc is usually straightforward: rest from overhead use of the arm; physiotherapy, in the form of short wave and exercises; and local injections of hydrocortisone and local anaesthetic. **The patient requires mild analgesics.**

4. Frozen shoulder – adhesive capsulitis – periarthritis. In this condition, which may be brought on by overuse, there is a widespread inflammatory reaction over the whole capsule with the formation of adhesions.

Fig. 9.24   Limitation of internal rotation and abduction in a 'frozen' shoulder.

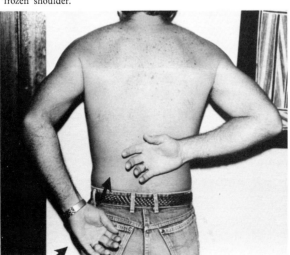

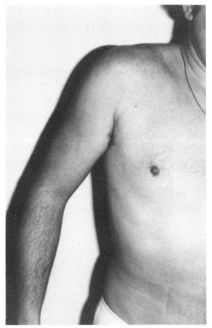

This patient has pain felt at the deltoid insertion with some radiation down the arm and up into the neck. There is rapid loss of shoulder movement (Fig. 9.24) and as the shoulder stiffens, the pain decreases. However the patient often is unable to sleep on the affected side. The stiffness may spontaneously resolve over a period of twelve months.

Treatment of this lesion depends on how much pain and stiffness is present. Pain is best treated by ice packs or heat. Stiffness is best treated by manipulation under an anaesthetic followed by physiotherapy. **This patient may require strong analgesia especially after a manipulation.**

Pain in the elbow region

Pain in the elbow can be:
   (a) Due to trauma;
   (b) Referred from the neck or shoulder; and
   (c) Due to local conditions.

Trauma around the elbow can be direct or indirect, and always warrants an X-ray. Fractures in this area are dealt with in Chapter 2. Note the problems of distinguishing epiphyses from fractures in children. The epiphyses are shown in detail in Figure 2.88.

If there is no fracture present, then the elbow may be simply bruised.

Pulled elbow

In children aged between one and four there is a condition called **'pulled elbow'**. This occurs when a little child is being held by the hand by an adult and is pulled up or along as he or she lags behind.

The 'pull' is such that the head of the radius, which does not yet have its cap formed, slips out of the orbicular ligament (Fig. 9.25).

The child will not use the arm and cries especially if the forearm is rotated. They hold the arm tightly to the body with the palm upwards.

Often, before they reach the consultant, the ligament clicks back on.

If you suspect this lesion from the history, then X-ray the elbow to make sure that there is no fracture and then replace the head with the following method – **take the child's hand and place his palm on the back of his neck.** You may not feel a click, but the proof that you now have the orbicular ligament in place is that you can rotate the forearm freely, and the child starts to use the arm.

Fig. 9.25 The reason for a 'pulled elbow' – slipping of the small head of the radius under the orbicular ligament.

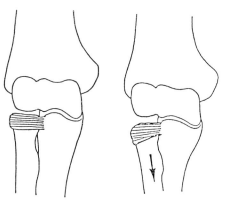

Local conditions

These can include arthritis in the elbow joint, and a much more common problem, epicondylitis.

Lateral epicondylitis or tennis elbow is by no means always associated with playing tennis. Many tennis players do have the condition. It is characterized by pain and local tenderness, often acute, over the lateral epicondyle. Gripping or forced flexion or extension of the wrist against resistance causes acute pain over the lateral side of the elbow. In workmen it is common for them to say they can't grip tools, and in the home people have difficulty picking up a phone book.

Treatment of this lesion can include the use of hydrocortisone injections, anti inflammatory drugs and, for tennis players, a special splint.

Medial epicondylitis is sometimes known as 'pitchers' elbow' for baseballers, and 'golfers' elbow' for golfers. The clinical picture is similar but the symptoms and the tenderness are on the medial side. Somehow the lesion does not seem to be as severe nor as persistent as lateral epicondylitis.

Pain in the wrist region

Most pain in the wrist has its origin in some form of trauma. Fractures around the wrist are dealt with in Chapter 2. **Remember that fractures of the scaphoid bone are notorious in that they often do not show up on the first X-ray.**

The message is clear. Any patient who has had a fall and who is tender over the radial side of the wrist must be X-rayed again at ten days, if the first film is clear.

Wrists can be bruised or strained, but this is a dangerous diagnosis until some weeks have passed and the second set of X-rays are normal – by that time the bruising or strain should have settled down.

Two other causes of pain are:
(a) De Quervain's disease
(b) Carpal tunnel syndrome

De Quervain's disease

This is a tendo-vaginitis of the thumb extensors and results in these tendons moving painfully in the fibrous sheath over the lateral side of the distal end of the radius. This gives the patient an acutely tender lump over the distal radius.

Finkelstein's test reproduces acute pain over the lump when you hold the end of the patient's thumb and ask him to extend the thumb.

Carpal tunnel syndrome

A burning pain, which often wakes the patient at night, and often tingling in the area of distribution of the median nerve characterises this condition. Patients say they wake after three hours of sleep and have to shake the hand and hang it down to get relief.

The syndrome is due to compression of the median nerve in the carpal tunnel and may be associated with tenosynovitis or fluid retention. It can occur after a fracture around the wrist, particularly if there is some malunion and therefore reduction in the size of the carpal tunnel.

Symptoms can be reproduced by having the patient sit for five to ten minutes with the wrists acutely flexed, and then applying gentle pressure over the median nerve.

Treatment will involve surgical decompression of the carpal tunnel and median nerve.

INDEX